CMA

STUDY GUIDE TEST PREP

2024-2025

Ace Your Medical Assistant Certification on the First Try | Tests | Q&A | Extra Content

Robert Cliven

EXLUSIVE EXTRA CONTENTS FOR YOU IN THE LAST CHAPTER!

I have recently decided to give **gifts** to all our readers. Yes, I want to provide you with the assistance that will help you with your study you will receive:

- **MP3 audio files** for you to listen to whenever and wherever you want!
- An eBook titled "**Medical Terminology for Health Careers.**"
- **NOW +600 flashcards with pictures** featuring "**Medical Terms**" for quick recall and enhanced comprehension.
- Digital version of this book
- **20** In-depth **Case Studies** offering real-world insights into patient safety, ethics, pain management, clinical communication, and care in varied settings.

Extra content for you

FLASHCARDS
with picture!

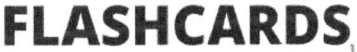
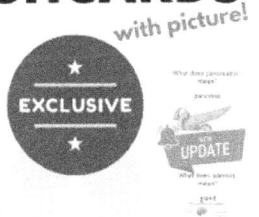

Extra content for you

AUDIOBOOK

Extra content for you

CASE STUDIES

You can track your progress and conveniently and interactively memorize the most important terms and concepts! Learn with printable flashcards or interactive flashcards on your device with **Anki APP or AnkiDroid!**

TABLE OF CONTENTS

INTRODUCTION

Welcome to the first chapter of your guide to the Certified Medical Assistant (CMA) Exam, an essential step in your journey towards becoming a vital healthcare team member. Aspiring CMAs like yourself are about to embark on a thrilling, challenging path that promises professional growth and a gratifying career in the medical field.

The CMA Exam is a rigorous, comprehensive test developed by the American Association of Medical Assistants (AAMA). This exam is designed to validate that you possess the clinical and administrative knowledge necessary to perform the job functions of a medical assistant in the United States.

Becoming a Certified Medical Assistant involves mastering diverse skills, from patient care and procedural assistance to administrative duties and office management. Hence, the CMA exam ensures you can uphold the highest professional standards while contributing to efficient, compassionate patient care.

The exam is divided into four key sections: **General, Administrative,** and **Clinical knowledge**, as well as an additional section on professional behavior. Each section covers various topics, ensuring a comprehensive evaluation of your readiness for the role of a CMA.

To better understand what lies ahead, let's break down these sections:

- **General:** This section assesses your understanding of medical terminology, anatomy, physiology, and pathology, along with your knowledge of patient rapport, communication, and professional behavior.
- **Administrative:** Here, your comprehension of medical reception, patient navigator duties, practice finances, and medical business practices will be evaluated.
- **Clinical:** This part of the exam focuses on your grasp of asepsis, infection control, assisting with examinations and treatments, patient education, and clinical pharmacology.
- **Professional Behavior:** This section evaluates your understanding of ethics, legal aspects of medicine, and protective practices, ensuring you're prepared to navigate complex scenarios while maintaining professionalism.

Passing the CMA Exam showcases your commitment to the medical assisting profession, which can significantly enhance your career prospects. Not only does it demonstrate your dedication to maintaining the utmost quality in patient care, but it also shows prospective employers your commitment to upholding the professional and ethical standards of the healthcare field.

This guide is designed to prepare you thoroughly for the CMA Exam. In the following chapters, we'll dive deep into each exam section, providing clear, concise information, practice questions, and strategies to help you tackle the exam confidently and successfully.

Remember, your journey to becoming a Certified Medical Assistant is not just about passing an exam. It's about cultivating a lifelong commitment to learning, improving, and delivering the best care possible. As you traverse this path, let this guide be your beacon, illuminating the way to a successful career as a Certified Medical Assistant.

Overview of the CMA Exam

As we delve deeper into the heart of the CMA Exam, let's explore its essential elements to ensure you comprehensively understand what awaits. This isn't just an examination—it's a crucial benchmark in your healthcare journey, assessing your readiness to shoulder significant responsibilities in a dynamic medical environment.

The CMA Exam, orchestrated by the American Association of Medical Assistants, is organized into three primary categories: General, Administrative, and Clinical. Each type scrutinizes distinct facets of medical assistance, forming a holistic evaluation of your proficiency. Let's delve into these categories further:

- **General:** This segment provides the foundation of your medical knowledge. It assesses your comprehension of basic biomedical sciences, including medical terminology, anatomy, physiology, and pathology. In addition, it evaluates your understanding of essential professional elements such as communication, medical law, and ethics. By exploring these topics, the exam ensures you're equipped with the fundamental knowledge integral to a medical assistant's role.

- **Administrative:** This category focuses on the crucial administrative aspects of medical assistance. From scheduling appointments and managing medical records to handling practice finances and insurance processes, this part gauges your capability to handle the day-to-day operations of a medical office. Through this section, the exam certifies your competence to perform administrative tasks efficiently, thereby ensuring the smooth functioning of a healthcare setting.

- **Clinical:** The Clinical category assesses your hands-on, practical skills necessary for patient care. This includes your understanding of asepsis, infection control, obtaining patient history, assisting with examinations and treatments, preparing and administering medications, and patient education. This section verifies your readiness to help physicians and care for patients in a clinical setting.

The CMA Exam encapsulates these wide-ranging categories to ensure you, as a future Certified Medical Assistant, can provide the highest standard of care to patients and support to physicians. It's a comprehensive evaluation designed to test your knowledge and skill and to affirm your commitment to the medical field.

As we navigate this guide, we will detail each category, providing you with in-depth knowledge, strategies, and practice questions. This is your path to successfully mastering the CMA Exam and stepping into a fulfilling career in healthcare. The journey might seem challenging, but remember that each step brings you closer to your goal. Stay tuned as we embark on this enriching journey together.

GENERAL MEDICAL KNOWLEDGE

Welcome to the second chapter of our guide, where we'll unfold the mysteries of the General Medical Knowledge section of the CMA Exam. This chapter will delve into the core scientific concepts that every medical assistant must master, providing you with the foundational information integral to your role in the healthcare environment.

The General Medical Knowledge section forms the bedrock of your medical understanding. This section emphasizes the essentials of biomedical sciences, encompassing anatomy, physiology, medical terminology, and pathology. Moreover, it includes essential professional elements like communication, medical law, and ethics, all vital to forming a well-rounded healthcare professional.

- **Anatomy and Physiology:** Understanding the human body, its systems, and how they function together is paramount for any healthcare professional. This segment tests your knowledge of the structure of the human body and its organs, the various bodily systems, their functions, and how they interrelate. To excel in this area, familiarize yourself with key concepts like cellular structure, bodily systems (such as the circulatory, nervous, and digestive systems), and the normal function and processes of these systems.

- **Medical Terminology:** You will constantly use unique medical terms as a medical assistant. Proficiency in medical terminology means you can effectively communicate with healthcare providers, patients, and insurance companies. This exam will assess your understanding of root words, prefixes, and suffixes commonly used in medicine. You should also be comfortable with abbreviations and symbols frequently used in patient records and prescriptions.

- **Pathology:** Pathology pertains to the study of diseases. It covers the cause of diseases, their effects on the body, symptoms, and the body's response to the disease process. By comprehending pathology, you can anticipate potential issues, understand a physician's diagnosis, and explain complex situations to patients in an accessible way. This aspect of your general medical knowledge is crucial to ensuring patients receive the best care possible.

- **Communication:** Excellent communication skills are critical in the healthcare field. You will often be the bridge between physicians and patients, ensuring clear and compelling exchanges. This exam portion will measure your ability to communicate orally and in writing, understand non-verbal cues, and use therapeutic communication techniques.

- **Medical Law and Ethics:** Ethical and legal knowledge is imperative to navigate healthcare. As a medical assistant, you will often face situations that require sound judgment based on legal and ethical principles. You must be familiar with patient rights, professional liability, and the legal implications of medical documentation. This part of the exam will test your ability to handle such situations professionally and ethically.

The General Medical Knowledge section of the CMA Exam is not just about rote memorization—it's about understanding how these elements weave together to form a comprehensive understanding of healthcare. As we dissect each aspect of this section in the following chapters, remember that this knowledge isn't only for passing an exam.

It is the groundwork for your success as a medical assistant, allowing you to provide compassionate, knowledgeable care for every patient you encounter. Approach this journey with curiosity and determination. The more deeply you understand these concepts, the more skilled and confident you will become as a healthcare provider.

As we venture into each topic, let's embrace the challenge and celebrate each step that brings us closer to becoming exceptional medical assistants.

Anatomy and Physiology

Diving deeper into the General Medical Knowledge section, we find ourselves at the heart of healthcare understanding - Anatomy and Physiology. This critical segment of the CMA exam assesses your comprehension of the human body's structure, its myriad functions, and the complex interplay between its various systems. A robust understanding of these concepts is vital for an efficient medical assistant.

- **Anatomy** is studying the body's structure—the bones, muscles, tissues, organs, and relationships. It's about understanding the 'where' and 'what' of our body. Each component has a specific location and role, from the minute cellular structures to the large organ systems. This knowledge helps you follow the physician's instructions accurately, administer medications correctly, and provide appropriate patient care.

As a medical assistant, you'll be expected to know the human body's major systems. These include the skeletal, muscular, nervous, endocrine, cardiovascular, respiratory, digestive, urinary, and reproductive systems. Each method has unique structures and functions you'll need to understand thoroughly. For instance, you should be familiar with how the skeletal system provides structural support and protection for the body or how the endocrine system regulates bodily functions through hormones.

- **Physiology**, on the other hand, delves into the 'how'—how our bodies function, how the organ systems work in harmony, and how our bodies adapt and respond to changes. The interrelationships between the organ systems are complex and dynamic, helping maintain balance or homeostasis, which is essential for survival. Understanding physiology allows you to recognize when something is not functioning as it should, a crucial skill in healthcare provision.

To illustrate, if you understand the cardiovascular system's physiology, you'll know that the heart pumps blood, carrying oxygen and nutrients to the body's cells. If this process is disrupted, cells don't receive what they need, leading to potential health complications. Your ability to comprehend such cause-and-effect relationships is a crucial indicator of your readiness to assist in patient care effectively.

It's important to note that while anatomy and physiology are separate fields of study, they are intrinsically connected. A thorough understanding of one enhances your comprehension of the other. Knowing the heart's structure (anatomy) will help you understand how it pumps blood throughout the body (physiology).

Similarly, understanding how the lungs exchange gases (physiology) is much easier if you know their structure (anatomy). By mastering anatomy and physiology, you're gaining theoretical knowledge and a fundamental understanding that will underpin your medical assisting career. It equips you with the tools to interpret what's happening beneath the skin, understand the root cause of a patient's symptoms, and provide appropriate support in the treatment process. As we delve further into these fascinating topics in the coming chapters, remember that this is the essence of healthcare. Each concept you learn, each connection you make, and each system you understand brings you one step closer to becoming an exceptional medical assistant ready to provide superior patient care. So, keep this enthusiasm alive, stay curious, and let's continue exploring the wonderful world of human anatomy and physiology together.

Medical Terminology

Next, we examine the intricate medical terminology—a specialized language health professionals use to communicate accurately and effectively. This lexicon of health-related terms forms the backbone of the healthcare communication system, allowing you to understand, interpret, and relay complex medical information. As a medical assistant, mastery of medical terminology is crucial for everyday interactions with patients, physicians, and other healthcare personnel.

- ***Medical terminology*** can initially appear complex, even daunting. Yet, it follows a systematic pattern, breaking down into smaller, understandable components—prefixes, roots, and suffixes. This standardized structure allows for an organized, universal approach to conveying healthcare-related information, reducing ambiguity, and enhancing clarity in communication.

- ***Root words*** are the core of medical terms, usually denoting a body part or a disease. They're often derived from Greek or Latin origins. For instance, the root 'cardi' pertains to the heart, while 'never' refers to nerves.

- ***Prefixes*** are added to the beginning of root words to provide additional context or specification. For example, 'hyper-' indicates excess or above average, while 'hypo-' signifies deficiency or below normal.

- ***Suffixe***d at the end of the root word, typically indicate a condition, procedure, or disease. 'itis,' for instance, denotes inflammation, and '-ectopy' implies removal or excision.

Through the combination of these components, you can decipher many medical terms. For instance, 'carditis' can be broken down into 'cardi-' (heart) and '-itis' (inflammation), signifying heart inflammation. Similarly, 'neurology' breaks down into near-' (nerve) and '-ology' (study of), indicating the breakdown of nerves.

In addition to these components, understanding commonly used medical abbreviations is vital to your medical terminology knowledge. In the fast-paced medical environment, abbreviations help convey information swiftly and efficiently. However, be cautious, as some abbreviations can have multiple meanings. Always consider the context to ensure correct interpretation.

Grasping medical terminology allows you to perform your duties as a medical assistant more effectively. It aids in interpreting physician's notes, transcribing medical records, explaining procedures to patients, and communicating with other healthcare professionals. More importantly, it helps reduce misunderstandings, a crucial factor in patient safety. The CMA Exam assesses your command over medical terminology, ensuring you can effectively navigate the healthcare environment. As you delve deeper into this language of medicine, you'll find it enriches your understanding and empowers you to contribute more meaningfully to patient care.

While learning medical terminology may seem formidable, remember it's about breaking down complex terms into simpler components. With consistent practice and study, you'll become more comfortable and proficient. Stay committed, and soon, these once unfamiliar terms will become second nature to you.

Remember that you are learning the very language of your profession—a language that enables you to connect, understand, and contribute to the world of healthcare. So, keep that spark of curiosity alive, and let's continue to explore this fascinating aspect of your medical assistant education.

Pathology and Disease Processes

As we continue our journey through the medical landscape, we arrive at an area of profound importance – Pathology and Disease Processes. This segment of your CMA Exam focuses on understanding the nature and causes of diseases, their effects on the body, and the body's responses to these conditions.

A medical assistant's grasp of pathology is essential as it facilitates accurate interpretation of symptoms, effective communication with other healthcare professionals, and meaningful support for patient care.

Pathology is the scientific study of diseases. It explores what causes a disease, how it progresses, its impact on the body, and the resulting symptoms or signs. This knowledge allows you to anticipate potential health issues, grasp a physician's diagnosis, and assist in managing patient health.

The study of disease processes involves understanding the sequence of biological events that lead to a diseased state. Diseases can stem from many factors, such as genetic abnormalities, infections, environmental influences, lifestyle habits, and aging. How these factors manifest as diseases is the crux of pathology.

Let's consider inflammation, a typical response to injury or infection. Recognizing the cardinal signs of inflammation—heat, redness, swelling, pain, and loss of function—can help identify a possible inflammatory condition. Similarly, understanding the typical stages of infection—from the incubation period to the disease's resolution—can aid in managing infectious diseases.

Furthermore, pathology extends to the examination of tissues and cells. Histopathology, for instance, studies the microscopic changes that diseases cause in body tissues, playing a critical role in disease diagnosis. While you may not perform these examinations as a medical assistant, understanding the basics can improve your ability to support the healthcare team.

Pathology also includes understanding systemic diseases—conditions that affect the body as a whole, such as diabetes or hypertension. Your grasp of these diseases' pathophysiology—how they disrupt normal bodily functions—will enhance your ability to assist in patient care and education. The CMA Exam's pathology section evaluates your ability to understand these disease processes, fostering an insightful medical assistant who can interpret clinical manifestations, comprehend diagnostic tests, and facilitate effective treatment strategies.

As we delve deeper into pathology, remember that understanding these disease processes is not just an academic exercise—it's about preparing you to support your patients better. It equips you with the knowledge to discern the potential implications of symptoms, empathize with the patient's condition, and explain complex health information in a manner patients can comprehend.

Learning pathology may seem challenging, but it's about piecing together the puzzle of the human body's response to disease. Stay engaged, keep questioning, and soon, the intricate tapestry of disease processes will unfold before you.

Remember that this knowledge equips you to contribute significantly to patient care. So, keep your curiosity kindled, and let's continue our journey into the fascinating world of pathology and disease processes.

Pharmacology

In healthcare, we find another pillar of critical importance - Pharmacology. This facet of the CMA Exam assesses your comprehension of medications, their effects on the body, and the principles governing their use. Pharmacology knowledge is indispensable for a medical assistant as it bolsters your capability to assist in patient care, ensuring safety and efficacy in medication management.

Pharmacology is the science of drugs. It explores how medications interact with the body's biological systems, affecting physiological functions. It's the art of healing, comfort, and often life-saving interventions. As a medical assistant, you'll frequently deal with medications, making your understanding of pharmacology both a responsibility and a necessity.

When exploring a medication, we consider several factors. These include the drug's generic and brand names, its therapeutic class, the conditions it's used to treat, and its mechanism of action - how it produces its therapeutic effect. Additionally, understanding a drug's route of administration, dosage forms, typical side effects, and potential drug interactions is integral to medication safety.

A foundational concept in pharmacology is the drug life cycle or pharmacokinetics - the process by which a drug is absorbed, distributed, metabolized, and eventually eliminated from the body. These dynamics influence the dosage and timing of a medication to ensure its optimal therapeutic effect. Pharmacodynamics is equally crucial - the study of how drugs affect the body. It examines the drug-receptor interaction and how it influences cell function. Pharmacodynamics helps predict a drug's therapeutic and adverse effects, assisting in choosing the most appropriate medication for a patient.

Pharmacology also covers the classification of drugs. Drugs are often grouped based on their therapeutic effect, such as analgesics for pain relief, antihypertensives for controlling high blood pressure, or antibiotics for treating bacterial infections. Understanding these classes enables you to appreciate the purpose behind a patient's medication regimen. Additionally, the study of pharmacology underscores the importance of the 'Five Rights' of medication administration - the right patient, the right drug, the correct dose, the correct route, and the right time. Adhering to these principles is paramount in preventing medication errors and safeguarding patient health.

As a medical assistant, your role in pharmacology extends beyond understanding medications. It involves educating patients about their medications, monitoring for adverse reactions, and advocating for patient safety. Your pharmacology knowledge forms the foundation of these tasks, promoting better patient outcomes.

The CMA Exam's pharmacology section challenges your grasp of these concepts, preparing you to handle medications competently and confidently. Pharmacology may seem like a vast and complex field, but it's about getting to know these therapeutic tools, understanding their benefits and risks, and optimizing their use for patient benefit.

Remember, each medication you learn, each drug interaction you understand, and each side effect you recognize is a step forward in your journey to becoming an exceptional medical assistant. It empowers you to assist in providing effective, safe, and patient-centered care.
So, let's embrace this learning journey, understand pharmacology's profound impact, and uncover your significant role in medication management. Your exploration of pharmacology is not just an academic endeavor—it's a path that leads you closer to becoming an indispensable part of the healthcare team

ADMINISTRATIVE ASPECTS

As we delve into the multi-faceted role of a Certified Medical Assistant (CMA), we can't overlook the profound significance of administrative aspects in healthcare. This portion of the CMA Exam evaluates your understanding of administrative tasks, emphasizing the need for skills beyond patient care. These range from managing medical records to handling insurance processes and contributing to the smooth operation of a healthcare facility.

When you picture a medical assistant, the first image that likely comes to mind is that of a healthcare professional aiding in clinical procedures. While that is indeed a significant part of the role, a medical assistant also serves as the backbone of administrative processes in healthcare facilities.

Medical assistants are the front-line representatives of a healthcare facility. They greet patients, schedule appointments, answer phone calls, and manage the reception area. Their professionalism, communication skills, and efficiency can significantly influence patients' perception of the healthcare facility.

A medical assistant's primary administrative responsibility is managing patient records. This involves accurately recording and updating patient information and ensuring the confidentiality and security of these records. Knowledge of Electronic Health Records (EHRs) systems is often essential, given their widespread use in modern healthcare facilities.

Medical assistants also play a significant role in insurance processes. They verify insurance information, submit claims, and may handle billing and coding tasks. This requires a sound understanding of health insurance policies, billing procedures, and medical codes for diagnoses and procedures.

In addition to these, medical assistants handle various other administrative tasks. These include ordering and inventory management of medical supplies, managing correspondence, and even assisting with the healthcare facility's marketing and public relations efforts.

A unique aspect of a medical assistant's administrative role is its function as a liaison. They bridge the gap between the patient and the healthcare team, the patient and their insurance provider, or even between different healthcare team members. This necessitates excellent communication skills and a patient-centric approach.

Now, why are these administrative tasks so crucial in healthcare? The reason is twofold. First, efficient administrative processes are critical to a healthcare facility's smooth and effective operations. They reduce wait times, prevent scheduling conflicts, and enhance patient experience. Second, they allow healthcare providers to focus on their primary duty - patient care. By relieving providers of administrative tasks, medical assistants enable them to spend more time with patients, improving the quality of care.

The Administrative Aspects section of the CMA Exam will challenge your understanding of these tasks and principles. It's not just about memorizing procedures or mastering software. It's about grasping the 'why' behind each task, appreciating the impact of your role, and understanding how you can contribute to a positive patient experience.

Remember, each patient interaction, record accurately updated, and successfully processed insurance claim contributes to patient satisfaction and quality care. As a medical assistant, you're supporting healthcare providers and enhancing patient care in ways that may not always be apparent but are nonetheless vital.

So, let's delve deeper into the administrative aspects of being a medical assistant. It explores the behind-the-scenes processes that keep a healthcare facility running smoothly and your role. It's about discovering how you can significantly impact patient care outside the clinical setting.

Medical Reception

As we navigate the administrative sphere of a medical assistant's responsibilities, let's look at one of the most pivotal roles: the Medical Reception. The medical receptionist often sets the tone for the patient's entire experience. The healthcare facility often forms its first and last impression through the eyes and actions of the receptionist.

Encompassing more than just greeting patients and answering phone calls, the role of a medical receptionist demands a delicate balance between interpersonal skills, organization, and an understanding of medical terminologies and systems. The medical receptionist juggles multiple responsibilities, serving as the face of the healthcare facility, the first point of contact, and an administrative powerhouse.

A vital duty of the medical receptionist is scheduling patient appointments. This includes managing a complex schedule, accommodating patient needs, and adjusting for unexpected changes, such as emergencies or cancellations. Efficient scheduling maximizes the provider's time, minimizes patient wait times, and allows for a smoother workflow in the healthcare facility.

Beyond scheduling, the receptionist is tasked with patient registration and updating patient records. This includes gathering necessary personal and insurance information from patients and ensuring it's accurately entered into the system. A well-organized patient database enhances patient care, improves communication, and expedites billing and insurance processes.

Notably, the medical receptionist manages communication within the healthcare facility. This involves taking and making phone calls, handling correspondence, and often liaising between patients and healthcare providers. Each communication touchpoint is an opportunity to provide exemplary service and foster a positive patient environment.

In addition to their patient-facing roles, medical receptionists often have several behind-the-scenes responsibilities. They manage the reception area, maintain office supplies, and may assist in basic financial tasks, like co-pay collection or billing queries. A clean, well-organized reception area enhances patient comfort and confidence in the healthcare facility, while efficient management of resources contributes to the facility's overall functionality.

As a medical receptionist, every interaction and task you perform has an impact. Your words can comfort a nervous patient, your organization can improve a healthcare provider's schedule, and your efficiency can enhance the overall functionality of the healthcare facility.

The Medical Reception section of the CMA Exam will evaluate your ability to perform these tasks. It will test your understanding of healthcare systems, administrative procedures, and communication skills. It's about proving your readiness to be the face of the healthcare facility, the first touchpoint in a patient's care journey. But remember, being a medical receptionist goes beyond passing an exam. It's about recognizing the difference you can make in a patient's experience. It's about understanding that your administrative role is integral to patient care.

As we explore the role of a medical receptionist, let's remember the power we hold in our hands. Each smile we give, each comforting word we say, each efficient action we take brings us closer to becoming not just a medical receptionist but a vital contributor to patient care.

Patient Navigator/Advocate

Before we delve into the specifics of the role of a patient Navigator/Advocate, let's take a moment to grasp the importance of this position. A patient's journey is often fraught with confusion and anxiety in healthcare. Amidst the labyrinth of medical terminologies, insurance protocols, and many specialist appointments, patients can feel lost and overwhelmed.

This is where the role of a Patient Navigator/Advocate becomes vital. As a Certified Medical Assistant (CMA), this role allows you to extend your assistance beyond immediate medical care, making a significant difference in a patient's healthcare journey. Let's unfold this crucial role and understand what it means to be a patient's navigator and advocate in the true sense.

Understanding the Role

In the modern healthcare system, a Certified Medical Assistant (CMA) often wears many hats, one of the most critical being the Patient Navigator or Advocate. This role focuses on guiding patients through the complex healthcare web as a beacon of support and guidance. A Patient Navigator/Advocate ensures that patients receive the necessary medical care and understand and navigate the healthcare system's intricacies.

Bridging the Gap

The role of a Patient Navigator/Advocate is to bridge the gap between the patient and the healthcare system. As a CMA, you are expected to guide patients through the labyrinth of healthcare, providing a compass for understanding medical terminology, procedures, and insurance processes. You become a crucial liaison, coordinating care and simplifying the complex.

Coordination of Care

A significant aspect of being a Patient Navigator/Advocate is care coordination. As a CMA, you may schedule appointments, follow up with specialists, ensure timely medical tests, and monitor treatment plans. This element requires a deep understanding of the healthcare system and a high level of organization. But more importantly, it requires empathy and compassion for the patients you're assisting.

Communication - The Key

Effective communication is the heart of patient advocacy. As a Patient Navigator/Advocate, your role requires explaining medical terms, procedures, and insurance claims in a language that patients can easily comprehend. This demystification of medical jargon can comfort patients, reducing their stress and empowering them to make informed decisions about their health.

Support Beyond Medical Care

The support offered by a Patient Navigator/Advocate often extends beyond medical care. You may find yourself assisting patients with insurance paperwork, exploring financial assistance options, or providing emotional support. Your role can be diverse, but the objective remains: to facilitate a patient's journey through healthcare, making it as smooth and stress-free as possible.

Preparation for the CMA Exam

The CMA exam's Patient Navigator/Advocate section will assess your understanding of these responsibilities. It will evaluate your communication skills, ability to coordinate care, knowledge of medical and insurance processes, and empathy and dedication to patient welfare.

However, remember that your role as a Patient Navigator/Advocate is not limited to passing an examination. It's about making a tangible difference in a patient's healthcare experience. It's about holding a patient's hand, metaphorically and sometimes literally, as they navigate the convoluted path of healthcare.

The Heart of Patient Advocacy

Being a Patient Navigator/Advocate is understanding that you hold a crucial role in patient care. You are the guide, the comforter, the organizer, and the translator. You help shape the patient's experience and their perception of healthcare.

As we delve deeper into the role of a Patient Navigator/Advocate, remember the fundamental mantra: it's about the patient. It's about their needs, their comfort, and their understanding. It's about making healthcare less daunting and much more compassionate. It's about making a difference, one patient at a time.

Medical Business Practices

The realm of healthcare extends far beyond the immediate medical care provided to patients. At the intersection of healthcare and business lies an essential, albeit less pronounced, aspect: Medical Business Practices. Although not directly involved in patient care, these practices form the backbone of a healthcare facility's smooth operation, ensuring that medical professionals can deliver timely and effective care to their patients.

As a Certified Medical Assistant (CMA), your role extends to these administrative areas, rendering you an invaluable asset in the healthcare industry. This section delves into the importance, elements, and implementation of Medical Business Practices, aiming to prepare you to handle the business side of healthcare adeptly.

The Intersection of Medicine and Business

At the juncture of healthcare and administration lies Medical Business Practices. While healthcare professionals prioritize providing high-quality medical care, well-structured business practices must be considered. These practices ensure the smooth operation of healthcare facilities, improving patient care and the institution's financial health.

As a Certified Medical Assistant (CMA), understanding Medical Business Practices is essential for efficiently managing a healthcare facility's non-clinical facets.

Importance of Medical Business Practices

The crux of Medical Business Practices lies in their importance to the seamless operation of healthcare institutions. By applying business principles, healthcare facilities can streamline their processes, improve patient satisfaction, and ensure efficient utilization of resources. This includes tasks such as scheduling patient appointments, maintaining medical records, billing, and insurance processing, which are all pivotal in a healthcare setting.

Scheduling and Organization

One of the first steps in effective medical business practices involves scheduling and organization. From managing patient appointments to coordinating staff schedules, a well-organized system is crucial for efficiently operating a healthcare facility. It not only improves staff productivity but also ensures that patients receive timely care.

Medical Records Management

Accurate and efficient management of medical records forms the backbone of any healthcare facility. Medical records hold vital patient information, which is necessary for delivering appropriate healthcare. Effective records management ensures timely access to these details and enhances the quality of care provided.

Billing and Insurance Processing

Navigating the world of healthcare finance, including billing and insurance processing, is another crucial aspect of medical business practices. A proficient understanding of these processes allows for a smoother patient experience and ensures the financial stability of the healthcare facility.

Compliance and Laws

Healthcare is a highly regulated industry with numerous compliance requirements. Adherence to laws and regulations protects both the institution and the patient. It ensures ethical practice, patient privacy, and quality of healthcare. Therefore, familiarity with healthcare laws and regulations is fundamental to medical business practices.

Preparation for the CMA Exam

The Medical Business Practices portion of the CMA exam assesses your knowledge in these areas. It evaluates your proficiency in scheduling, organization, records management, billing, insurance processing, and law compliance. A thorough understanding of these practices equips you to contribute significantly to efficiently running any healthcare facility.

The Role of a CMA in Medical Business Practices

As a CMA, you are a linchpin in Medical Business Practices. You ensure that the business side of healthcare runs smoothly, thus enabling doctors to focus on providing quality patient care. Your role contributes to the patient experience, healthcare quality, and the institution's financial health, making you an invaluable asset in the healthcare industry.

Remember, as we delve into the depths of Medical Business Practices, the goal is not merely about passing an examination but becoming well-equipped to manage the non-clinical aspects of a healthcare institution effectively. It's about ensuring the wheels of healthcare keep turning smoothly, and in doing so, you help deliver the best possible patient care.

Establishing Patient Medical Records

Creating and managing patient medical records are integral to the healthcare delivery system. These records are more than just a collection of medical histories and treatment plans; they are crucial in ensuring continuity and quality in patient care.

A well-managed medical record is a treasure trove of patient information, allowing healthcare providers to make informed decisions and offer personalized care. As a Certified Medical Assistant (CMA), understanding how to establish patient medical records is paramount in your role.

The Crucial Role of Medical Records

A patient's medical record serves as healthcare providers' primary information source. It describes the patient's medical history, diagnostic tests, treatment plans, progress notes, and other vital information. This comprehensive document facilitates cohesive, effective, and personalized medical care.

Establishing Medical Records: The Initial Step

Establishing a medical record begins with the patient's first encounter with the healthcare provider. The basic information - the patient's personal details, the reason for the visit, and medical history - is collected during this visit. This is the foundation upon which the medical record is built, and its accuracy is essential for effective healthcare delivery.

Inclusion of Essential Medical Information

Following the initial data collection, it is necessary to populate the medical record with more specific medical information. This includes details of any diagnoses, prescribed medications, surgical history, allergies, immunizations, and any other relevant healthcare information. Every subsequent visit, diagnosis, and treatment plan adds to this record, creating a comprehensive account of the patient's medical journey.

Maintaining Confidentiality and Ensuring Compliance

CMAs must strictly adhere to the Health Insurance Portability and Accountability Act (HIPAA) guidelines in handling patient medical records. This law ensures the protection of patient information and stipulates strict standards for the handling of medical records. A CMA must ensure compliance with these regulations to protect the patient's privacy and the integrity of the healthcare institution.

The Role of Technology: Electronic Health Records (EHRs)

Most healthcare facilities have transitioned from paper records to Electronic Health Records (EHRs) in today's digital age. These digital records facilitate easy access to patient information, enhance communication among healthcare providers, and enable effective patient care management. Understanding the workings of EHR systems is vital for a CMA to manage patient records efficiently.

The Cornerstone of Quality Healthcare

Properly establishing and managing patient medical records cannot be overstated. These records are pivotal in providing effective, personalized care to patients. They foster communication among healthcare providers and provide valuable data for research and quality improvement initiatives.

As a CMA, your role in establishing and maintaining these records is essential in the delivery of quality healthcare. As we move forward, remember the intricacies of medical records management go beyond passing an examination. It's about acquiring skills that enhance patient care, streamline healthcare processes, and contribute significantly to the healthcare delivery system.

Scheduling Appointments and Practice Finances

As a Certified Medical Assistant (CMA), your role extends beyond patient care and into administrative responsibilities. Two such crucial aspects are the **scheduling of appointments and managing practice finances**. A well-coordinated appointment system ensures the smooth flow of patients, maximizing efficiency. Simultaneously, understanding practice finances is vital to the economic health and sustainability of the medical practice. This section takes a deep dive into these interconnected roles.

The Art of Scheduling

Appointment scheduling is often likened to a balancing act. CMAs have to ensure the smooth flow of patients without overbooking or under booking the healthcare provider's time. The aim is to reduce patient waiting times while ensuring that healthcare providers have enough time to provide quality care to each patient.

An effective scheduling system considers the reason for the visit, estimating the time required for different types of appointments. Emergencies, new patient visits, and routine follow-ups require an additional time allocation. Moreover, CMAs should also consider the healthcare provider's availability and preferences.

Electronic appointment scheduling has become the norm with the rise of digital solutions. It provides convenience to patients and efficiency to healthcare practices. Understanding the operation of such systems is an essential skill for CMAs.

Managing Practice Finances: An Overview

On the other hand, managing practice finances involves a broad spectrum of tasks, including but not limited to billing, insurance claims, budgeting, and financial reporting. A firm grip on these financial aspects allows a medical practice to sustain itself, ensuring it can continue providing patient care.

As a CMA, you may be involved in preparing patient bills and processing payments. Understanding the basics of medical coding and billing is essential for this task. Accurate billing ensures that the practice is compensated appropriately for the services provided.

Handling insurance claims is another vital aspect. CMAs need to understand the different types of insurance plans, the process of filing claims, and how to follow up on unpaid claims. Navigating this process efficiently ensures timely compensation and reduces financial strain on the practice.

Budgeting and financial reporting, while usually handled by practice managers or financial officers, are still essential for a CMA to understand. A basic understanding of these processes allows CMAs to contribute to financial discussions and make informed decisions about practice operations.

The Interplay Between Scheduling and Finances

At first glance, scheduling and finance may seem distinct. However, they are closely interlinked. Effective scheduling maximizes the use of resources, improving the practice's financial efficiency. For instance, reducing no-shows and cancellations, achieved through effective scheduling, can significantly improve a practice's financial health.

CMAs: The Backbone of a Smooth-Running Practice

In conclusion, CMAs play a crucial role in maintaining the administrative harmony of a healthcare practice. The ability to schedule appointments effectively and understand practice finances is vital to your role as a CMA.

While it can seem daunting, these tasks become second nature with practice. As a CMA, your role in these administrative aspects makes you an essential part of the healthcare team, ensuring a smoothly running approach focusing on what matters most – patient care.

CLINICAL ASPECTS

The role of a Certified Medical Assistant (CMA) is an intricate blend of patient care, administrative tasks, and technical prowess. A significant portion of this responsibility lies in the domain of clinical care, where CMAs are instrumental in supporting healthcare providers and ensuring patients receive top-notch care. This chapter will explore the various facets of the CMA's clinical roles and responsibilities.

Patient Interaction: More Than Just Healthcare

Interaction with patients forms the bedrock of a CMA's clinical duties. This interaction begins the moment a patient steps into the healthcare facility. As a CMA, you'll be the first point of contact, making you responsible for creating a comforting environment that can alleviate the patient's anxieties.
From here, you will record patient histories, understand their concerns, and even explain procedures. Effective communication is essential throughout these interactions to ensure patients are informed, comfortable, and prepared for their visit.

Assisting in Examinations and Procedures

CMAs often assist healthcare providers during physical examinations and medical procedures. This can range from preparing the exam room and arranging necessary medical instruments to aiding the healthcare provider. In some cases, CMAs may also perform simple functions under the healthcare provider's supervision.

Collecting and Preparing Laboratory Specimens

Another key aspect of a CMA's clinical responsibilities involves handling laboratory specimens. Depending on the state laws and the practice's requirements, CMAs may collect samples like blood, urine, or tissues. Once collected, these samples are analyzed in-house or prepared for sending to an external laboratory. Understanding the correct collection, storage, and transport methods is crucial to ensure the accuracy of test results.

Performing Basic Laboratory Tests

In many healthcare facilities, CMAs perform basic laboratory tests. This includes analyzing urine samples for routine urinalysis or performing rapid tests for conditions like strep throat or influenza. Accurate performance and interpretation of these tests are fundamental for the appropriate treatment of patients.

Administering Medications

Administering medications as directed by a healthcare provider is another pivotal clinical duty of CMAs. This requires a comprehensive understanding of the medications, including their uses, dosages, routes of administration, and potential side effects. Moreover, CMAs must also know the legal and ethical considerations when administering medications.

Patient Education and Follow-Up

Patient education forms a significant part of a CMA's responsibilities. CMAs often instruct patients about medications, diet, lifestyle modifications, and follow-up care. They may also conduct follow-up calls to check on patients' progress and address any concerns they might have.

Infection Control and Safety Measures

In the healthcare setting, maintaining a safe environment is paramount. CMAs play an essential role in implementing infection control measures, which include proper hand hygiene, safe disposal of medical waste, sterilization of medical instruments, and adhering to personal protective equipment guidelines.

The Scope of Clinical Practice

The scope of a CMA's clinical duties can vary greatly depending on state laws and the type of medical practice. Some CMAs may specialize in a particular area of clinical practice, such as pediatrics or geriatrics, while others may work in a general practice where they handle various clinical tasks.

In conclusion, the clinical role of a CMA is multifaceted and dynamic. It intertwines technical skills, medical knowledge, and compassionate care, forming the heart of patient care. As a CMA, your clinical work doesn't just support healthcare providers but directly impacts patients, making your role invaluable in healthcare delivery.

Patient Interview, Examination Room Techniques

In the bustling world of healthcare, Certified Medical Assistants (CMAs) often act as the backbone, supporting the functions of the medical team in myriad ways. Their role spans various aspects of patient care, and two significant areas include the Patient Interview and Examination Room Techniques. While distinct in their requirements, these areas are interconnected in their ultimate goal: providing comprehensive, compassionate, and efficient patient care. In the subsequent sections, we delve into the intricate processes, protocols, and the art of communication required in both these domains to ensure an optimal healthcare experience for patients.

Patient Interview: Building Bridges of Communication

An effective patient interview forms the backbone of a successful healthcare encounter. It is the initial touchpoint where a Certified Medical Assistant (CMA) gathers essential information about the patient's current health concerns, medical history, lifestyle, and overall well-being.

Interviewing a patient requires a deep sense of empathy and excellent communication skills. The objective is to foster a safe and open environment where patients feel comfortable sharing their health concerns and personal information. This is often achieved by demonstrating respect for the patient's experiences, validating their feelings, and showing a genuine interest in their well-being. Firstly, establishing rapport is the cornerstone of an effective patient interview. This includes providing a warm greeting, maintaining eye contact, and engaging in small talk to put the patient at ease. Remember, you set the tone for the patient's entire healthcare experience, so a friendly, non-judgmental approach is crucial.

Subsequently, you must collect the patient's chief complaint or the primary reason for their visit. This should be in the patient's own words and noted accurately in the patient's medical record. Following this, gather a detailed history of the present illness (HPI). Ask open-ended questions to encourage the patient to describe their symptoms, their onset, duration, frequency, and any factors that aggravate or alleviate these symptoms.

Next, delve into the patient's past medical history, including any chronic illnesses, hospitalizations, surgeries, and allergies. Also, remember to ask about their family and social history, including lifestyle habits such as smoking, alcohol use, diet, and exercise, as these can greatly influence a person's health. The medication history is another essential component of the patient interview.
Obtain a comprehensive list of the patient's current medications, including prescription drugs, over-the-counter medicines, and any supplements they may take. To conclude the interview, summarize the information gathered, and allow the patient to clarify or add any additional information. This verifies the data's accuracy and will enable patients to feel heard and involved in their care.

Examination Room Techniques: The Stage for Quality Healthcare

Once the patient interview is complete, the next step in a CMA's clinical role involves examination room techniques. This encompasses many tasks, from preparing the examination room to assisting during the examination.

The process starts even before the patient enters the examination room. As a CMA, you must ensure the room is clean, organized, and stocked with necessary supplies. This includes examination gloves, gowns, drapes, and any specific equipment the healthcare provider might require, like a stethoscope, otoscope, or sphygmomanometer.

When the patient arrives, guide them into the examination room and provide clear instructions about what they need to do. If the examination requires the patient to undress or wear a gown, ensure they understand this process while maintaining their comfort and privacy.

During the examination, your role might involve handing instruments to the healthcare provider, holding and comforting the patient, or performing tasks such as taking the patient's vital signs or documenting findings. Your precise duties may vary depending on the healthcare provider's needs, the type of examination, and the patient's condition.

Sterilizing instruments post-procedure and disposing of medical waste correctly is an integral part of the examination room technique. It ensures the safety of both patients and healthcare providers by preventing the spread of infections. Moreover, a CMA might also need to clean and restock the examination room after each patient. This includes general cleaning tasks and involves ensuring that equipment is functioning correctly, reporting any issues to the relevant department, and maintaining an inventory of supplies.

In conclusion, effective examination room techniques ensure that healthcare procedures are conducted smoothly and efficiently. As a CMA, you play a critical role in ensuring the healthcare provider has everything they need and that the patient is comfortable and well cared for during the examination. With these practices, you contribute significantly to the quality of healthcare services provided.

Collecting and Processing Specimens

The science of medicine requires data, which often comes from within us in the form of various bodily specimens. The collection and processing of these specimens is a fundamental part of the work performed by Certified Medical Assistants (CMAs), and it's essential for the diagnoses, treatment plans, and overall management of a patient's health.

Mastering the techniques of specimen collection begins with understanding the variety of specimens that can be collected, including but not limited to blood, urine, sputum, stool, and tissue samples. Each instance can reveal much information about a patient's health status, but only if the model is collected and processed correctly.

Taking blood, for example, demands precision and professionalism. Every step matters from the moment you verify the patient's identity and explain the procedure to the point where you apply the tourniquet, select the appropriate needle, and puncture the vein. The same goes for urine collection, whether a routine urinalysis or a clean-catch midstream specimen. Each process has its specifics that must be meticulously followed to avoid cross-contamination or erroneous results. Moreover, processing specimens is as crucial as collecting them. It involves a series of tasks, including labeling, preparing for analysis, and storing or shipping the models as necessary. Mislabeling can result in significant errors in patient care, while improper preparation can compromise test results. It's a CMA's responsibility to follow the protocols meticulously and manage any unforeseen circumstances that may arise.

For example, blood samples must be centrifuged to separate serum or plasma from blood cells, while urine samples for a culture test must be refrigerated promptly if not processed within an hour of collection. Familiarity with the onsite laboratory equipment and a sound knowledge of the guidelines for specimen processing become key factors for CMAs in this regard. Notably, safety is paramount throughout these procedures. CMAs must adhere to the Occupational Safety and Health Administration (OSHA) standards to protect themselves and their patients from possible exposure to infectious materials. They must use personal protective equipment, implement biohazard waste disposal methods, and promote a clean environment.

Equally important is communication. CMAs often have to explain the procedures to patients and address their concerns and sometimes even their fears. Comforting a needle-phobic patient, for example, might involve talking them through the process, using a smaller needle, or employing a distraction technique. Therefore, the essence of effective specimen collection and processing lies in the blend of technical skills, safety measures, and interpersonal communication.

It's a testament to the complexity of the healthcare field that something as seemingly straightforward as collecting and processing specimens can entail so many elements. But for CMAs, who are the crucial link between the patients and the medical team, mastering these tasks is part of their commitment to patient care. They work behind the scenes, often unheralded, but their role is invaluable in facilitating accurate diagnoses and effective treatments. Their attention to detail and commitment to their role enhance patients' trust in healthcare, making them genuinely unsung healthcare heroes.

Emergency Management/Basic First Aid

Emergency management and basic first aid are cornerstones of patient care in the healthcare setting. They form the first line of defense when a life-threatening situation arises. For Certified Medical Assistants (CMAs), these skills are vital as they often act as the initial responders before a patient sees a doctor or other healthcare providers.

Emergency Management: Making the Right Call

In an emergency, seconds can mean the difference between life and death. CMAs need to be trained to assess and respond to emergencies swiftly and appropriately. Emergency management starts with recognizing the situation. A patient's sudden chest pain, difficulty breathing, severe bleeding, or unconsciousness are clear signs of a medical emergency. CMAs must stay calm, promptly inform the physician, and ensure the emergency medical team is alerted if necessary.

Proper patient assessment plays a crucial role. Checking vital signs, keeping track of changes in the patient's condition, and documenting these observations accurately all feed into the medical team's intervention strategies. Moreover, CMAs should be equipped to use automated external defibrillators (AEDs) and administer cardiopulmonary resuscitation (CPR) if required.

Basic First Aid: Immediate Care, Maximum Impact

Although seemingly simple, basic first aid can profoundly affect a patient's well-being. The primary goal is to keep the patient stable until more advanced medical treatment can be administered. Simple actions, like placing an unconscious patient in recovery to keep their airway clear, can make a significant difference in their condition.

Understanding the basics of wound care is another crucial aspect. Whether it's a minor cut or a more severe wound, CMAs should know how to clean the wound, apply the appropriate dressing, and when to recognize the signs of infection. In the case of burns, different degrees require different approaches. First-degree burns can typically be managed with cool water and a sterile dressing. However, more severe burns require immediate medical intervention to manage pain and prevent infection. CMAs should know to differentiate the burn levels and provide the proper initial care.

Communication in Emergency Situations

Communication is key in emergency situations. CMAs must reassure and inform patients about their care while communicating clearly and concisely with other healthcare professionals. This aids in better decision-making and facilitates a smoother, more effective response. Furthermore, in emergency scenarios, CMAs should understand the Incident Command System (ICS) principles. This structured approach to handling emergencies improves response efficiency and ensures that every staff member understands their role and responsibilities.

In conclusion, emergency management and basic first aid knowledge are essential for CMAs. They serve as the first response line in situations requiring immediate attention. By mastering these skills, CMAs play an invaluable role in improving patient outcomes and maintaining a high standard of care in their healthcare facilities.

Pharmacology

As an integral component of the healthcare system, pharmacology—the study of drugs and their effects on the human body—is a key area of expertise for a Certified Medical Assistant (CMA). Understanding this field is essential for safe and effective medication administration, patient education, and monitoring for potential side effects or adverse reactions.

Unraveling the Complex World of Drugs

Many drugs exist in the medical landscape, each with unique characteristics, modes of action, and potential interactions. CMAs should familiarize themselves with the major drug classes, including but not limited to antibiotics, antihypertensives, antidiabetics, anticoagulants, and analgesics. Understanding these classes and their common representatives allows CMAs to anticipate their effects, potential side effects, and any special administration considerations.

Administration and Dosage

One of the primary roles a CMA may undertake is medication administration. The 'Five Rights' of medication administration—right patient, drug, dose, route, and time—are non-negotiables in any healthcare setting. Mistakes in these areas can have serious consequences, even for simple medications.

Dosages vary widely between patients, depending on age, weight, kidney function, and other health conditions. An awareness of these variables and a sound understanding of the drug itself will help CMA avoid dosing errors and potential harm.

Drug Interactions and Contraindications

Drugs can interact with each other, with food, or with specific medical conditions, and these interactions can alter the effects of a drug. Some interactions can enhance the desired therapeutic effect or unwanted side effects. Others can reduce the drug's effectiveness, potentially leading to treatment failure.

Knowing the everyday interactions of widely used drugs and recognizing when to raise concerns can be instrumental in patient safety. The same applies to contraindications—specific conditions or factors that make a particular medication or treatment inadvisable. This knowledge enables CMAs to be an additional safety net in the healthcare team.

Patient Education and Advocacy

CMAs often find themselves in a position to educate patients about their medications. This task involves explaining in layperson's terms what the drug does, why it is being given, how it should be taken, and what side effects may occur. This education is crucial in ensuring patient compliance with their medication regimen. Furthermore, CMAs can act as patient advocates, observing and reporting adverse drug effects. By maintaining a vigilant eye and open communication lines with patients, CMAs can help ensure medications serve their healing purpose without causing undue harm.

Pharmacology forms a significant part of a CMA's training and everyday role. It's a complex, ever-evolving field that demands continual learning and careful attention. From drug knowledge and administration to patient education and advocacy, CMAs are crucial in ensuring safe and effective medication use in their healthcare settings. Their contributions in this domain directly impact patient health outcomes, highlighting the importance of their role and the necessity of their expertise.

Patient Education and Communication

Patient education and communication are foundational aspects of healthcare delivery. A Certified Medical Assistant (CMA) often serves as a critical communication link between healthcare professionals and patients, requiring proficiency in educational principles and effective communication strategies.

Patient Education: Empowering through Knowledge

Patient education is about more than explaining a diagnosis or treatment plan. It's about empowering patients with the knowledge to make informed decisions about their health, understand their responsibilities, and actively participate in their care.

One of the primary areas of patient education involves medication instruction. CMAs need to explain to patients what each medication is for, how and when to take it, potential side effects to watch for, and any necessary dietary or lifestyle adjustments.

Health education also extends to disease prevention and health promotion. CMAs may discuss diet and nutrition, exercise, stress management, and preventive screenings. They may also teach self-care skills to patients with chronic diseases, helping them to manage their condition effectively.

In all these areas, a successful patient education approach requires clear, concise information presented in a manner that respects the patient's health literacy level.

The Art of Communication

Good communication is key to successful patient education. But what does this entail in a healthcare setting?

Firstly, it requires active listening. When CMAs take the time to listen to a patient's concerns and questions, they show respect for the patient's experiences and build a trusting relationship. Active listening also helps CMAs to understand the patient's perspective, providing insight that can guide educational efforts.

Secondly, effective communication means speaking clearly and using language the patient can understand. Medical jargon should be replaced with simple, everyday language. Visual aids, printed materials, and demonstrations can supplement verbal explanations and help to ensure understanding.

Thirdly, communication involves checking for understanding. This is often achieved through the "teach-back" method, where patients are asked to explain what they have been told in their own words. This method allows CMAs to assess whether the information has been understood and clarify misconceptions.

Lastly, effective communication means being sensitive to a patient's emotions and showing empathy. This sensitivity can create an environment where patients feel comfortable asking questions and sharing concerns.

The Power of Non-Verbal Communication

Non-verbal cues like body language, facial expressions, and tone of voice can convey as much information as words. By maintaining eye contact, adopting an open posture, and using an empathetic manner, CMAs can reinforce their comments and help to create a positive communication environment.

Navigating Cultural Differences

CMAs may encounter patients from different cultural backgrounds in an increasingly diverse society. Understanding and respecting cultural differences in health beliefs and practices is crucial for effective communication and education. This cultural competence can avoid misunderstandings and foster a collaborative healthcare relationship.

Whether explaining a medication regimen, teaching a new self-care skill, or addressing a patient's concerns, patient education and communication are at the heart of a CMA's role. By mastering these skills, CMAs can facilitate better health outcomes, enhance patient satisfaction, and contribute to a more effective healthcare system. As the healthcare landscape continues to evolve, the importance of patient education and effective communication only grows, highlighting their crucial role in a CMA's toolbox.

Effective Communication

Effective communication is more than a tool in healthcare—it's a lifeline that connects all parties involved, fosters healing relationships, and facilitates optimal patient care. Certified Medical Assistants (CMAs) serve as a primary point of contact and are crucial in maintaining this lifeline.

The Cornerstones of Effective Communication

Effective communication is built on clarity, respect, empathy, and active listening.

- **Clarity** ensures that the information shared is precise, easy to understand, and free from medical jargon. It involves using language that matches the patient's level of comprehension and health literacy.

- **Respect** underpins each interaction. It involves respecting the patient's rights, values, preferences, and autonomy, recognizing that each patient actively participates in their healthcare journey.

- **Empathy** refers to the ability to understand and share the feelings of another. In a healthcare setting, empathetic communication can help patients feel understood and supported, promoting a therapeutic relationship.

- **Active listening** involves fully concentrating on, understanding, responding to, and remembering a patient's words. It is key to building trust, fostering rapport, and understanding the patient's perspective.

Verbal and Non-Verbal Communication

Verbal communication is the use of words to transfer information. In a healthcare context, this can involve explaining a diagnosis, providing instructions for medication use, or discussing care plans.

However, communication is about more than just the spoken or written word. Non-verbal communication—such as facial expressions, body language, and tone of voice—also plays a significant role. For instance, an open posture can convey approachability, steady eye contact can show attentiveness, and a calm, gentle tone of voice can provide reassurance.

Effective Communication Across Different Mediums

In the digital age, communication extends beyond face-to-face interactions. CMAs may need to communicate with patients via phone, email, patient portals, or telemedicine platforms. Each medium has its unique aspects that require careful navigation. For example, telephone or telemedicine communication lacks the visual cues available in face-to-face communication, requiring clear verbal communication and attentive listening.

Overcoming Communication Barriers

Healthcare communication can face numerous barriers—differences in language or culture, low health literacy, fear or anxiety, and physical disabilities such as hearing loss. CMAs must be equipped to navigate these challenges, using tools like medical interpreters, educational materials, simple language, and assistive technologies to ensure clear communication.

Communication Skills in Practice

Effective communication is not just about individual interactions—it also impacts broader areas of healthcare practice. For example, it is crucial to ensure informed consent, where patients need clear, comprehensive information to make informed decisions. It also plays a role in conflict resolution, where open, respectful dialogue can help resolve disagreements and maintain positive team dynamics.

The Impact of Effective Communication

Effective communication in healthcare can lead to improved outcomes, including increased patient satisfaction, better adherence to treatment plans, decreased patient anxiety, and improved health status. Furthermore, it can lead to more efficient healthcare delivery and better interprofessional collaboration.

In conclusion, effective communication is a vital skill in the toolbox of any CMA. It requires ongoing learning and practice but can lead to profound improvements in patient care and professional satisfaction. As healthcare becomes increasingly patient-centered, the role of effective communication will only continue to grow, highlighting the importance of mastering this skill for any aspiring CMA.

Patient Education Principles

Patient education plays a vital role in the healthcare system, empowering patients to actively participate in their own care and make informed decisions about their health. As a Certified Medical Assistant (CMA), it is crucial to understand and implement practical patient education principles. This section will explore key strategies and considerations for delivering comprehensive patient education in a medical setting.

Assessing Patient Needs

Before initiating any patient education, assessing the individual's needs, including their medical condition, literacy level, cultural background, and personal preferences, is essential. This assessment helps tailor the educational approach to meet the patient's unique requirements.

Clear Communication

Effective patient education relies on clear and concise communication. Use plain language that patients can easily understand, avoiding jargon and complex medical terminology. Use visual aids, such as anatomical diagrams, charts, and models, to enhance comprehension and facilitate discussion.

Health Literacy

Health literacy refers to a person's ability to obtain, process, and understand basic health information. As a CMA, assessing patients' health literacy levels and adapting educational materials is crucial. Simplify complex concepts, provide written materials at an appropriate reading level, and encourage patients to ask questions to ensure comprehension.

Individualized Approach

Recognize that each patient is unique and requires an individualized approach to education. Tailor educational content to match the patient's specific condition, treatment plan, and personal circumstances. When developing educational strategies, consider age, language proficiency, cultural beliefs, and socioeconomic status.

Active Engagement

Engage patients actively in the learning process to enhance their understanding and retention of information. Encourage questions and provide opportunities for patients to demonstrate their knowledge through verbal or written explanations. Utilize interactive teaching methods, such as role-playing or hands-on demonstrations, to reinforce key concepts.

Multimodal Teaching

Employ a variety of teaching methods to cater to different learning styles. Some patients prefer visual learning, while others benefit from auditory or kinesthetic approaches. To accommodate diverse learning preferences and enhance patient engagement, utilize multimedia resources, such as videos or interactive online tools.

Reinforcement and Follow-up

Patient education should be a process rather than a one-time event. Reinforce critical information during subsequent visits and provide written materials for patients to refer to at home. Encourage patients to actively participate in their care by providing additional resources, such as reliable websites or support groups, for further learning and support.

Cultural Sensitivity

Recognize and respect cultural differences when delivering patient education. Be mindful of cultural beliefs, practices, and health disparities that may influence the patient's understanding and acceptance of medical information. Incorporate culturally sensitive materials and adapt teaching methods to ensure inclusivity and effective communication.

CMAs can foster a collaborative and empowering healthcare environment by adhering to these patient education principles. Effective patient education promotes better health outcomes, increased patient satisfaction, and a strengthened partnership between patients and healthcare providers. As a CMA, your role in patient education is integral to improving overall patient care and promoting health literacy within the community.

Cultural Competence

In the diverse healthcare landscape, cultural competence is essential for Certified Medical Assistants (CMAs). Cultural competence refers to understanding, respecting, and effectively communicating with individuals from diverse cultural backgrounds. It involves recognizing and addressing patients' unique beliefs, values, practices, and needs, ultimately fostering a more inclusive and patient-centered approach to care. This section will explore the importance of cultural competence in healthcare and provide strategies for CMAs to enhance their cultural competence skills.

Importance of Cultural Competence in Healthcare

Improved Communication and Trust

Cultural competence facilitates effective communication between healthcare providers and patients from different cultural backgrounds. When CMAs demonstrate an understanding and respect for cultural differences, patients feel heard, valued, and understood. This leads to establishing trust, which is vital for effective healthcare delivery.

Enhanced Patient Engagement and Participation

Cultural competence encourages patients to engage in their healthcare decisions actively. When CMAs take the time to learn about their patient's cultural beliefs, practices, and values, they can incorporate these factors into the care plan. CMAs empower patients to make informed decisions and take ownership of their health by involving patients in their care.

Reduction of Health Disparities

Cultural competence plays a crucial role in reducing health disparities among diverse populations. By understanding the cultural factors that may influence health behaviors and access to care, CMAs can develop culturally appropriate and responsive interventions. This helps bridge the gap in healthcare outcomes between different cultural groups.

Strategies to Enhance Cultural Competence

Self-Reflection and Awareness

Developing cultural competence starts with self-reflection. CMAs should examine their biases, assumptions, and beliefs about different cultures. This introspection helps increase self-awareness and lays the foundation for understanding and respecting cultural diversity in healthcare.

Cultural Humility

Cultural humility involves recognizing that one's own cultural background may limit their understanding of others. CMAs should approach interactions humbly, acknowledging that they continually learn from patients and their diverse experiences. This mindset promotes open-mindedness and a willingness to adapt to different cultural perspectives.

Knowledge of Cultural Practices

CMAs should proactively seek knowledge about the cultural practices and beliefs prevalent among their patients. This includes understanding cultural norms related to health, communication styles, dietary preferences, traditional healing practices, and religious or spiritual beliefs. By familiarizing themselves with these aspects, CMAs can provide culturally sensitive care.

Effective Communication

Effective communication is essential for cultural competence. CMAs should use clear and plain language, avoiding medical jargon or complex terminology that may confuse patients. It is also important to be attentive to non-verbal cues and body language, as these can vary across cultures and convey different meanings.

Respect for Privacy and Modesty

Respecting cultural norms regarding privacy and modesty is crucial in promoting patient comfort and trust. CMAs should be mindful of practices related to physical touch, eye contact, and gender-specific care preferences. CMAs can create a safe and respectful patient environment by adapting their approach to align with cultural expectations.

Collaboration and Teamwork

Cultural competence extends beyond individual interactions with patients. CMAs should collaborate with a diverse healthcare team, including interpreters, cultural liaisons, and other professionals who can provide insights into specific cultural practices. By working together, the healthcare team can ensure that patient care is comprehensive and culturally sensitive.

Continuing Education

Cultural competence is an ongoing learning process. CMAs should actively seek professional development and education opportunities on cultural competence topics. This may involve attending workshops, participating in cultural competency training programs, or engaging in self-study to deepen their understanding of diverse cultures and healthcare disparities.

Feedback and Evaluation

CMAs should seek patient, colleague, and supervisor feedback to evaluate their cultural competence skills. This feedback can help identify areas for improvement and guide further professional development. Regular self-assessment and reflection are essential to enhance cultural competence continuously.

In conclusion, cultural competence is vital for CMAs in providing patient-centered care. By embracing cultural diversity, practicing effective communication, and respecting the beliefs and values of patients from various cultural backgrounds, CMAs can foster trust, engagement, and better health outcomes. Cultural competence is an ongoing journey requiring self-reflection, knowledge acquisition, and collaboration with diverse healthcare teams. CMAs contribute to a more inclusive and equitable healthcare system by integrating cultural competence into their practice.

Legal and Ethical Considerations

The role of a Certified Medical Assistant (CMA) extends beyond mere medical support—it also encompasses critical elements of legal and ethical conduct within a healthcare setting. Understanding the complexities of these considerations is pivotal for successful and responsible practice. This chapter delves into these critical aspects, providing a comprehensive look at how CMAs must navigate the dynamic landscape of medical ethics and law.

Understanding Legal Boundaries

The Importance of Scope of Practice

As a CMA, it's crucial to understand the legal boundaries that define your 'scope of practice.' Each state defines this uniquely, dictating the tasks that a CMA can perform. Crossing these boundaries knowingly or unknowingly may lead to allegations of medical malpractice or negligence. Thus, maintaining awareness of your defined role and duties is a foundational legal compliance element.

Confidentiality and Health Information Privacy

The Health Insurance Portability and Accountability Act (HIPAA) plays a significant role in a CMA's practice. It mandates the protection of patient privacy and the confidentiality of health information. Breaching these regulations can lead to severe legal consequences. Consequently, CMAs must always be HIPAA compliant, from secure data management to maintaining patient confidentiality.

Ethical Considerations

Patient Autonomy and Informed Consent

In healthcare, ethical principles like patient autonomy—i.e., a patient's right to self-determination—are sacrosanct. CMAs must respect and uphold this principle. One of the essential aspects of patient autonomy is informed consent, which involves explaining procedures, potential risks, and benefits to patients, ensuring they have all the information necessary to make decisions about their care.

Nonmaleficence and Beneficence

Two further foundational ethical principles in healthcare are nonmaleficence, meaning "no harm," and beneficence, which urges medical practitioners to act in the patient's best interest. These principles remind CMAs of their obligation to safeguard patients from harm and prioritize their well-being.

Conflict Resolution

Legal and ethical considerations sometimes appear conflicting, creating moral dilemmas. Knowing how to navigate these situations is essential, often requiring a balance of professional guidelines, personal morals, and legal obligations. Regular consultation with peers, mentors, and institutional ethics committees can provide valuable guidance in such instances.

Cultural Competence and Sensitivity

A CMA's role often includes interacting with diverse patient populations. Therefore, displaying cultural competence and sensitivity is crucial, respecting each patient's unique cultural, social, and personal values. Failure to do so may lead to suboptimal care and result in legal and ethical violations.

The role of a CMA is fraught with challenges. It involves more than just proficient medical assistance—it demands a thorough understanding and commitment to legal and ethical standards.

While rules and regulations may vary, the ethical considerations—patient autonomy, nonmaleficence, beneficence—are universal. A CMA, therefore, must be adept at navigating the medical landscape and the intricate web of legal and ethical considerations in the quest to provide quality patient care.

Regulatory Guidelines for Certified Medical Assistants

In addition to the ethical and legal considerations previously outlined, CMAs must adhere to regulatory guidelines set forth by federal, state, and professional bodies. These rules provide a robust framework for healthcare practices, guiding CMAs in delivering quality patient care while mitigating legal risks.

Federal Regulations

Health Insurance Portability and Accountability Act (HIPAA)

HIPAA forms a cornerstone of patient information security. This federal regulation safeguards the privacy of patients, governing how medical information is stored, shared, and accessed. CMAs should be familiar with HIPAA's Privacy Rule, which protects individuals' medical records and other health information, and its Security Rule, which sets standards for protecting health information held or transferred electronically.

Occupational Safety and Health Administration (OSHA)

OSHA regulations ensure safety in the workplace by maintaining standards for infection control, hazard communication, and emergency preparedness. CMAs must adhere to these guidelines to provide patients and healthcare workers with a safe and healthy environment.

State Regulations

While federal regulations apply nationwide, state regulations can vary significantly. CMAs should understand the specifics of their state's guidelines regarding their practice, including but not limited to:

Medical Practice Acts

These state laws regulate the practice of medicine, including defining the scope of practice for medical assistants. They may determine what CMAs can and cannot do within their roles, such as administering medications, taking vital signs, or assisting in minor surgeries.

State-specific Patient Privacy Laws

Some states may have privacy laws that extend beyond HIPAA's requirements, providing even more stringent protection for certain types of health information. Adherence to these laws is critical to avoid penalties and ensure respect for patient privacy.

Professional Regulatory Guidelines

Professional organizations such as the American Association of Medical Assistants (AAMA) also provide regulatory guidelines and codes of conduct. FOR EXAMPLE, the AAMA's Code of Ethics and Creed sets forth principles of honesty, respect, and professionalism, offering a roadmap for CMAs to navigate ethical and moral situations.

Infection Control and Sterilization Guidelines

In addition to OSHA's broad guidelines, the Centers for Disease Control and Prevention (CDC) provides specific recommendations for infection control in healthcare settings. These guidelines cover essential procedures such as hand hygiene, use of personal protective equipment, sterilization of medical instruments, and disposal of medical waste.

The Importance of Continuing Education

Regulatory guidelines can and do change, making it imperative for CMAs to commit to continuous learning. Many states and professional organizations require ongoing education as part of certification renewal. These courses can keep CMAs up-to-date on the latest legal, ethical, and professional standards, ensuring their practice remains at the forefront of patient safety and care.

Navigating the complex world of regulatory guidelines is critical to a CMA's role. By remaining knowledgeable and compliant with these rules, CMAs can ensure they provide the highest level of care and protect themselves, their patients, and their workplaces from potential legal and ethical violations.

Medical Law and Ethics

Medical Law

Medical law is the backbone of healthcare practice, providing a firm structure of rules and regulations that healthcare professionals, including Certified Medical Assistants (CMAs), must adhere to. The primary objective of medical law is to ensure safe, efficient, and ethical healthcare services.

Understanding Medical Malpractice

One of the most critical aspects of medical law is medical malpractice. CMAs must recognize what constitutes malpractice, such as negligence, to avoid legal complications. Failure typically involves a healthcare professional failing to provide the standard of care that a reasonably competent professional would have provided in a similar situation, harming the patient.

Informed Consent

Informed consent is another crucial component of medical law. Before any medical procedure, a CMA must ensure patients understand the procedure's purpose, potential benefits and risks, and alternative options. Failing to obtain informed consent can lead to legal implications, including allegations of battery or negligence.

Mandatory Reporting

Certain circumstances require CMAs to report specific information, such as suspected child abuse, certain infectious diseases, or threats of self-harm. Failing to adhere to mandatory reporting laws can lead to legal consequences and, in some cases, compromise patient safety.

Medical Ethics

While medical law provides the legal framework for healthcare, medical ethics is the moral compass guiding CMAs' actions and decisions. It involves making judgments about what is right or wrong, good or bad, in a healthcare setting.

Beneficence and Nonmaleficence

Beneficence, the principle of doing good, urges CMAs to act in ways that benefit patients. On the other hand, nonmaleficence, often summarized as "do not harm," compels CMAs to avoid causing harm to patients. These principles work together, reminding CMAs of their primary responsibility to promote patient health and well-being while minimizing damage.

Autonomy and Respect for Persons

The principle of autonomy underscores the importance of respecting patients as individuals capable of making informed decisions about their health. This principle closely ties with informed consent, which is a legal requirement and an ethical obligation to respect patient autonomy.

Justice

The principle of justice in healthcare refers to treating all patients equitably, regardless of factors such as age, race, gender, socioeconomic status, or disease state. CMAs must strive to ensure resources are distributed fairly, and all patients are given equal healthcare access and treatment opportunities.

Confidentiality

Confidentiality is another ethical principle that plays a significant role in healthcare. All patients have a right to privacy regarding their health information. CMAs must uphold this right, only sharing patient information when necessary and appropriate, such as for treatment purposes or when legally mandated.

In conclusion, the interplay of medical law and ethics shapes the roles and responsibilities of CMAs. By understanding and adhering to these principles, CMAs can navigate the complexities of healthcare, providing the highest standard of care to their patients while maintaining professionalism and legal compliance.

PRACTICE TEST

Clinical Workflow: Patient Intake and Discharge

1. **What is the first step a CMA should take in patient intake?**
   - **A.** Assess the patient's vital signs
   - **B.** Conduct a physical exam
   - **C.** Verify the patient's identity
   - **D.** Schedule the next appointment

2. **What information must a CMA collect from a new patient during intake?**
   - **A.** patient's contact details and medical history
   - **B.** Patient's current medications
   - **C.** Patient's insurance details
   - **D.** All of the above

3. **Which of the following is not typically a CMA's responsibility during patient discharge?**
   - **A.** Giving discharge instructions
   - **B.** scheduling follow-up appointments
   - **C.** Prescribing medications
   - **D.** Reviewing the care plan

4. **When scheduling a follow-up appointment, what key factor should be considered?**
   - **A.** patient's availability
   - **B.** Provider's availability
   - **C.** The nature and urgency of the follow-up
   - **D.** All of the above

5. **Which document should a patient sign to consent to treatment?**
   - **A.** Medical history form
   - **B.** Insurance form
   - **C.** Informed Consent form
   - **D.** Discharge summary

6. **A patient has forgotten their insurance card at home. What should a CMA do?**
   - **A.** Reschedule the appointment
   - **B.** Proceed with the appointment and ask the patient to bring it next time
   - **C.** Call the insurance company to verify coverage
   - **D.** Deny treatment until proof of insurance is provided

7. **At what point should patients be educated about their privacy rights under HIPAA?**
   - **A.** During discharge
   - **B.** After treatment
   - **C.** During the first visit
   - **D.** When requested by the patient

8. **Who is typically responsible for developing a patient's care plan?**
   - **A.** The patient
   - **B.** The CMA
   - **C.** The physician
   - **D.** The patient's insurance company

9. **Which of the following is an essential step in the discharge process?**
   A. Giving the patient a copy of their medical record
   B. Making sure the patient understands their care plan
   C. Scheduling the next patient's appointment
   D. Updating the patient's insurance information

10. **When is a patient's discharge summary typically completed?**
    A. Before the patient's appointment
    B. During the patient's appointment
    C. After the patient's appointment
    D. At the time of the next appointment

11. **When conducting patient intake, which vital signs should a CMA typically check?**
    A. Heart rate
    B. Respiratory rate
    C. Blood pressure
    D. All of the above

12. **What important task should be completed if a patient is transferred to another healthcare provider?**
    A. Updating the patient's medical history
    B. Sending a complete patient health record to the new provider
    C. Informing the insurance company
    D. Getting the patient's consent for the transfer

13. **A CMA can provide medical advice to a patient.**
    A. True
    B. False

14. **What's the appropriate action if a patient doesn't attend their scheduled appointment?**
    A. Reschedule the appointment
    B. Charge a no-show fee
    C. Reach out to the patient to inquire about their absence
    D. Dismiss the patient from the practice

15. **During patient discharge, what critical information should a CMA relay to the patient regarding their prescribed medication?**
    A. Price of the medication
    B. How to administer the medication
    C. The pharmaceutical company's reputation
    D. All of the above

16. **In the case of a minor, who can provide consent for a medical procedure?**
    A. The minor, themselves
    B. The minor's guardian or parent
    C. The minor's teacher
    D. Any adult present

17. **What is the role of a CMA in the case of an emergency in the clinic?**
    A. Perform surgery
    B. Administer first aid and call for emergency medical services
    C. Console, the patient's family
    D. Prescribe medication

18. **In terms of medical records, what does the acronym PHI stand for?**
    A. Patient Health Information
    B. Private Health Insurance
    C. Personal Health Index
    D. Public Health Initiative

19. **What is the correct procedure if a patient arrives late for an appointment?**
    A. Cancel the appointment
    B. Rush through the appointment to make up for lost time
    C. Reschedule the appointment
    D. Proceed with the appointment but inform the patient that it may need to be cut short

20. **Who typically explains the discharge summary to the patient?**
    A. The physician
    B. The CMA
    C. The pharmacist
    D. The insurance company representative

21. **What is the primary purpose of a patient intake form?**
    A. To provide a record of the patient's insurance
    B. To document the patient's symptoms and reason for the visit
    C. To obtain the patient's medical history and demographic information
    D. To keep a record of the patient's payment history

22. **What does a CMA typically do if a patient cannot comprehend the discharge instructions?**
    A. Dismiss the patient immediately
    B. Hand the patient a written copy of the instructions
    C. Explain again using simpler terms or provide additional resources
    D. Ask the patient to find someone who can understand the instructions

23. **What is the primary consideration when scheduling follow-up appointments?**
    A. The CMA's convenience
    B. The clinic's operating hours
    C. The patient's medical necessity
    D. The availability of medical supplies

24. **During patient intake, a CMA must confirm the patient's identity. What is the most common way to do this?**
    A. Ask the patient to verify their name and date of birth
    B. Ask the patient for a fingerprint
    C. Take a photo of the patient for the records
    D. Ask the patient to provide their Social Security number

25. **How should a CMA handle a patient who refuses a recommended treatment during discharge?**
    A. Insist on the treatment
    B. Document the refusal in the patient's medical record
    C. Reschedule the appointment
    D. Cancel the patient's medical insurance

26. **In what format should discharge instructions be provided to the patient?**
    A. Verbal instructions only
    B. Written instructions only
    C. Both verbal and written instructions
    D. Instructions were given to a family member or caregiver only

27. **What should a CMA do if they notice a patient's medical history discrepancy during intake?**
   - **A.** Ignore it
   - **B.** Alter the medical record to match the patient's account
   - **C.** Discuss the discrepancy with the patient for clarification
   - **D.** Report the patient to their insurance company

Safety and Infection Control

1. **Which regulatory agency mandates the use of Universal Precautions in healthcare settings?**
   - **A.** OSHA
   - **B.** FDA
   - **C.** CDC
   - **D.** WHO

2. **Which of the following is the correct method for handling biohazardous waste?**
   - **A.** Putting it in a regular trash bin
   - **B.** Flushing it down the toilet
   - **C.** Placing it in a designated, clearly marked container
   - **D.** Leaving it in the patient's room

3. **What does the term "asepsis" mean?**
   - **A.** Presence of pathogens
   - **B.** Absence of disease
   - **C.** Absence of pathogens
   - **D.** Presence of disease

4. **Which of these is a Standard Precaution in infection control?**
   - **A.** Using gloves when touching blood, body fluids, secretions, and excretions
   - **B.** Wearing a mask only when the patient has a known airborne disease
   - **C.** Washing hands only after direct patient contact
   - **D.** Cleaning equipment only when visibly soiled

5. **In which situation should a CMA use an N95 respirator?**
   - **A.** When taking vital signs
   - **B.** When dealing with a patient with an airborne disease, like TB
   - **C.** When cleaning the clinic
   - **D.** During administrative duties

6. **What is the primary purpose of using Personal Protective Equipment (PPE)?**
   - **A.** To protect the patient from the healthcare worker
   - **B.** To protect the healthcare worker from potential exposure to infectious materials
   - **C.** To ensure the healthcare worker looks professional
   - **D.** To avoid the need for hand hygiene

7. **What is the first step in responding to a chemical spill in the clinic?**
   - **A.** Clean it up immediately
   - **B.** Inform the patient
   - **C.** Notify your supervisor or the responsible personnel
   - **D.** Leave the clinic

8. **How should sharps (like needles) be disposed of in a clinical setting?**
   - **A.** In a regular trash bin
   - **B.** In a designated sharps container
   - **C.** In a recycling bin
   - **D.** Down the sink

9. **What is the most effective method of preventing the spread of germs in a healthcare setting?**
   - **A.** Wearing gloves
   - **B.** Wearing a mask
   - **C.** Hand hygiene
   - **D.** Using an air purifier

10. If a CMA gets a needlestick injury, what should they do first?
    A. Continue with their duties
    B. Wash the area with soap and water
    C. Squeeze the wound to promote bleeding
    D. Apply a bandage

11. What is the correct sequence of donning Personal Protective Equipment (PPE)?
    A. gown, mask/respirator, goggles/face shield, gloves
    B. Mask/respirator, gloves, gown, goggles/face shield
    C. Gloves, mask/respirator, gown, goggles/face shield
    D. Goggles/face shield, gown, mask/respirator, gloves

12. What is the main principle of surgical asepsis?
    A. Only sterilized equipment and supplies must be used
    B. Hand hygiene is not required
    C. Gloves are not necessary
    D. Infectious waste can be disposed of in a regular trash bin

13. What type of fire extinguisher should be used on an electrical fire?
    A. Water extinguisher
    B. Foam extinguisher
    C. CO2 extinguisher
    D. Wet chemical extinguisher

14. What is the term for a disease that can be transmitted from person to person?
    A. Communicable
    B. Noncommunicable
    C. Incurable
    D. Chronic

15. Which of these is NOT a bloodborne pathogen?
    A. HIV
    B. Hepatitis B
    C. Tuberculosis
    D. Hepatitis C

16. Which type of isolation precaution should be used for patients with diseases like measles or chickenpox?
    A. Contact precautions
    B. Droplet precautions
    C. Airborne precautions
    D. Standard precautions

17. How often should hand hygiene be performed in a healthcare setting?
    A. Only at the beginning and end of a shift
    B. Only after direct contact with a patient
    C. Before and after every patient interaction, after touching potentially contaminated surfaces, and before putting on and after removing PPE
    D. Only when hands are visibly soiled

18. What does "MSDS" stand for in a healthcare setting?
    A. Medical Sterilization and Disinfection System
    B. Material Safety Data Sheet
    C. Medical Safety and Disease Standards
    D. Material Storage and Disposal System

19. What is the recommended procedure if a healthcare worker gets splashed in the eye with potentially infectious material?

A. Wipe the eye with a tissue
B. Rinse the eye with water or saline for at least 15 minutes
C. Continue with duties and monitor for symptoms
D. Apply an eye ointment and cover it with a patch

20. **What is one of the main reasons for double-bagging medical waste?**
    A. To ensure the waste is not visible
    B. To provide an extra layer of protection against leaks or tears
    C. To make the waste heavier
    D. To color-code the waste for easier sorting

21. **Which of the following statements about autoclaving is false?**
    A. Autoclaving can sterilize medical instruments
    B. Autoclaving works by using steam under pressure
    C. Autoclaving requires specific temperature and pressure conditions
    D. Autoclaving effectively cleans instruments but does not sterilize them

22. **What does the color 'red' signify in a healthcare setting about waste management?**
    A. General waste
    B. Recyclable materials
    C. Infectious waste
    D. Chemical waste

23. **What is the primary purpose of the Safety Data Sheet (SDS) in a healthcare setting?**
    A. To list the hospital's operating hours
    B. To provide important information about potential hazards and safety precautions for handling, storing, and transporting chemicals
    C. To outline the healthcare center's organizational hierarchy
    D. To document patients' medical histories

24. **If a healthcare worker is exposed to a patient's blood, what is the first thing they should do?**
    A. Continue with their duties
    B. Immediately wash the exposed area with soap and water
    C. Wait for the end of their shift to clean the area
    D. Apply a bandage to the exposed area

25. **What does 'PPE' stand for in a healthcare context?**
    A. Professional Practice Evaluation
    B. Personal Protective Equipment
    C. Patient Privacy Ethics
    D. Physician Practice Essentials

26. **Which type of hepatitis is a vaccine available for?**
    A. Hepatitis A and B
    B. Hepatitis B and C
    C. Hepatitis C and D
    D. Hepatitis D and E

27. **Which of the following should not be done when using a fire extinguisher?**
    A. Pull the pin
    B. Aim low
    C. Squeeze the handle
    D. Spray in a circular motion

Procedures/Examinations

1. **Where would the healthcare professional most likely listen to detect aortic regurgitation during a physical examination?**
   A. The second intercostal space at the right sternal border
   B. The second intercostal space at the left sternal border
   C. The fifth intercostal space at the midclavicular line
   D. The fifth intercostal space at the right sternal border

2. **A Certified Medical Assistant is asked to perform a Snellen Test. What does this test assess?**
   A. Hearing acuity
   B. Visual acuity
   C. Balance
   D. Reflexes

3. **A patient reports experiencing vertigo. Which type of examination is best suited to investigate this complaint?**
   A. Otoscopic examination
   B. Neurological examination
   C. Cardiac examination
   D. Respiratory examination

4. **What does an optimistic Murphy's sign indicate during a physical examination?**
   A. Appendicitis
   B. Gallbladder disease
   C. Kidney infection
   D. Pancreatitis

5. **Which of the following positions is most suitable for a rectal examination?**
   A. Supine
   B. Prone
   C. Sims'
   D. Trendelenburg

6. **When should a tourniquet be removed during a venipuncture procedure?**
   A. Immediately after the needle is inserted
   B. Just before the needle is withdrawn
   C. After the last tube has been filled and before the needle is withdrawn
   D. After the needle is withdrawn

7. **What type of suture material would be most suitable for suturing a high-tension area like a joint?**
   A. Absorbable sutures
   B. Non-absorbable sutures
   C. Adhesive strips
   D. Staples

8. **What is the primary purpose of an electrocardiogram (ECG)?**
   A. To evaluate lung function
   B. To assess brain activity
   C. To measure blood pressure
   D. To monitor heart rhythms

9. In a Pap smear, cells are most commonly collected from which part of the female reproductive system?
    A. Uterus
    B. Ovaries
    C. Cervix
    D. Fallopian tubes

10. What is the medical term for a procedure that involves examining a body cavity using a flexible tube with a light and a camera?
    A. Angiography
    B. Endoscopy
    C. Bronchoscopy
    D. Radiography

11. Where would a healthcare provider palpate during a physical exam to assess the liver?
    A. Right upper quadrant
    B. Left upper quadrant
    C. Right lower quadrant
    D. Left lower quadrant

12. What examination method is typically used to assess a patient's joint mobility and muscle strength?
    A. Auscultation
    B. Percussion
    C. Palpation
    D. Inspection

13. Which type of patient positioning allows the best examination of the posterior thorax and lungs?
    A. Supine
    B. Prone
    C. Lithotomy
    D. Sims'

14. Where should the swab be applied when conducting a throat swab for strep throat?
    A. The roof of the mouth
    B. The inner cheek
    C. The back of the throat
    D. The tongue

15. What does a positive Romberg sign indicate?
    A. Inner ear dysfunction
    B. Vision impairment
    C. Musculoskeletal abnormality
    D. Respiratory issue

16. What is the purpose of a Holter monitor?
    A. To measure blood pressure over 24 hours
    B. To monitor heart rhythm continuously over 24 hours
    C. To monitor glucose levels continuously over 24 hours
    D. To measure lung function over 24 hours

17. In an adult patient, which vein is most commonly used for venipuncture?
    A. Radial vein
    B. Femoral vein
    C. Median cubital vein
    D. Great saphenous vein

18. **What is the most appropriate site for intramuscular injection in an adult?**
    A. Deltoid muscle
    B. Ventrogluteal muscle
    C. Vastus lateralis muscle
    D. All of the above

19. **Which medical imaging technique uses radio waves and a strong magnetic field to produce detailed images of the inside of the body?**
    A. X-ray
    B. Ultrasound
    C. Computed tomography (CT)
    D. Magnetic resonance imaging (MRI)

20. **What diagnostic tool primarily measures the oxygen saturation level in a patient's blood?**
    A. Sphygmomanometer
    B. Pulse oximeter
    C. Spirometer
    D. Stethoscope

21. **Which physical examination technique might be used in a patient suspected of having appendicitis?**
    A. McBurney's point of tenderness
    B. Percussion of Traube's space
    C. Palpation of the costovertebral angle
    D. Measurement of JVP

22. **Which imaging modality best visualizes soft tissue injuries such as ligament tears?**
    A. X-Ray
    B. CT Scan
    C. MRI
    D. PET Scan

23. **Which substance is typically measured to assess kidney function during a comprehensive metabolic panel?**
    A. Glucose
    B. Creatinine
    C. Albumin
    D. Bilirubin

24. **What position should a patient be in to evaluate jugular venous pressure best?**
    A. Supine
    B. Sitting upright
    C. Sims' position
    D. Trendelenburg position

25. **Which of the following is the primary purpose of a bronchoscopy?**
    A. To assess the function of the heart
    B. To visualize the bronchi and diagnose lung conditions
    C. To evaluate blood flow in the arteries
    D. To measure brain activity

26. **When should the blood samples be collected when performing a glucose tolerance test?**
    A. Just before the glucose drink is consumed
    B. Immediately after the glucose drink is consumed
    C. At intervals after the glucose drink is consumed
    D. Both A and C

27. **What medical device is used to monitor a patient's heart rate and rhythm over a more extended period, often 24 hours or more?**
    - **A.** Electroencephalogram (EEG)
    - **B.** Electrocardiogram (ECG)
    - **C.** Holter monitor
    - **D.** Pacemaker

28. **What is the primary purpose of a spirometry test?**
    - **A.** To evaluate kidney function
    - **B.** To evaluate lung function
    - **C.** To assess the structure of the heart
    - **D.** To assess glucose metabolism

29. **Which diagnostic procedure would be most helpful in diagnosing a bone fracture?**
    - **A.** CT scan
    - **B.** MRI
    - **C.** Ultrasound
    - **D.** X-ray

Pharmacology

1. **Which classification of drugs is primarily used to reduce high blood pressure?**
    A. Diuretics
    B. Antidepressants
    C. Antifungals
    D. Anticoagulants

2. **What is the primary therapeutic effect of opioid medications?**
    A. Reduce inflammation
    B. Relieve pain
    C. Treat bacterial infections
    D. Control seizures

3. **Which medication would likely be prescribed for a patient with a bacterial infection?**
    A. Ibuprofen
    B. Amoxicillin
    C. Furosemide
    D. Metformin

4. **What is the primary purpose of administering a diuretic?**
    A. To increase the heart rate
    B. To increase urine output
    C. To decrease urine output
    D. To decrease the heart rate

5. **Which of the following routes of administration would be most appropriate for a rapid response in an emergency?**
    A. Oral
    B. Sublingual
    C. Intravenous
    D. Topical

6. **What term describes a severe, potentially life-threatening allergic reaction that can occur after taking a medication?**
    A. Anaphylaxis
    B. Myocardial infarction
    C. Stroke
    D. Asthma attack

7. **Which medication treats patients with type 2 diabetes by helping their bodies use insulin more effectively?**
    A. Beta-blockers
    B. Anticoagulants
    C. Metformin
    D. ACE inhibitors

8. **Which classification of drugs is most often used to treat anxiety disorders?**
    A. Benzodiazepines
    B. Statins
    C. Beta-blockers
    D. Diuretics

9. **What is the primary action of anticoagulant medications?**
    A. Lower blood pressure
    B. Prevent blood clot formation
    C. Reduce pain
    D. Control blood sugar levels

10. **Which of the following drugs is a nonsteroidal anti-inflammatory drug (NSAID)?**
    A. Ibuprofen
    B. Paracetamol
    C. Morphine
    D. Digoxin

11. **What medication is commonly used to treat symptoms of depression?**
    A. Lithium
    B. Fluoxetine
    C. Metformin
    D. Losartan

12. **Which medication is used to reverse the effects of an opioid overdose?**
    A. Naloxone
    B. Fentanyl
    C. Methadone
    D. Morphine

13. **What drug is used for its antiviral properties to treat HIV?**
    A. Digoxin
    B. Zidovudine
    C. Alprazolam
    D. Furosemide

14. **Which class of drugs is typically used to treat arrhythmias?**
    A. Antifungals
    B. Antipyretics
    C. Antiarrhythmics
    D. Anticoagulants

15. **Which type of medication can lead to the risk of stomach ulcers if used long-term?**
    A. Beta-blockers
    B. Statins
    C. NSAIDs
    D. ACE inhibitors

16. **What medication is typically administered to asthmatic patients to prevent an asthma attack?**
    A. Metformin
    B. Albuterol
    C. Zidovudine
    D. Diazepam

17. **What type of medication is often used to control high cholesterol levels?**
    A. ACE inhibitors
    B. Benzodiazepines
    C. Statins
    D. Beta blockers

18. **Which of these drugs is used to control seizures in epileptic patients?**
    A. Metformin
    B. Levothyroxine
    C. Carbamazepine
    D. Hydrochlorothiazide

19. **Which drug can be used to treat both hypertension and benign prostatic hyperplasia (BPH)?**
    A. Tamsulosin
    B. Sildenafil
    C. Prednisone
    D. Losartan

20. **What is the primary therapeutic action of antiemetic drugs?**
    A. To prevent or reduce nausea and vomiting
    B. To reduce pain
    C. To lower blood glucose levels
    D. To fight bacterial infections

21. **Which medication would be appropriate to treat hypothyroidism?**
    A. Metformin
    B. Albuterol
    C. Levothyroxine
    D. Warfarin

22. **Which type of medication is typically used in the treatment of glaucoma?**
    A. Proton pump inhibitors
    B. Beta-blockers
    C. Benzodiazepines
    D. Opioids

23. **Which medication is used to treat allergic reactions?**
    A. Diphenhydramine
    B. Acetaminophen
    C. Lisinopril
    D. Metoprolol

Legal and Ethical Issues

1. **What federal law in the United States requires the confidentiality of patient health information?**
   A. HIPAA
   B. EMTALA
   C. CLIA
   D. FERPA

2. **What principle of medical ethics requires healthcare providers not to harm?**
   A. Autonomy
   B. Beneficence
   C. Non-maleficence
   D. Justice

3. **Which of the following is an example of a breach of patient confidentiality?**
   A. Discussing a patient's condition with another healthcare provider involved in their care
   B. Leaving a patient's medical records open in a public area
   C. Requiring patients to sign in when they arrive for an appointment
   D. Asking a patient for their health history

4. **If a patient refuses treatment, what ethical principle supports the patient's right to make this decision?**
   A. Autonomy
   B. Beneficence
   C. Justice
   D. Non-maleficence

5. **Which law prevents healthcare providers from denying emergency care due to a patient's inability to pay?**
   A. EMTALA
   B. HIPAA
   C. CLIA
   D. FERPA

6. **What would be the most appropriate action if a medical assistant witnesses a coworker falsifying a patient's record?**
   A. Confront the coworker directly
   B. Ignore it as it's not their responsibility
   C. Report it to a supervisor or the practice's compliance officer
   D. Make a note of the incident for personal records

7. **Which ethical principle refers to fairness in medical treatment and the distribution of healthcare resources?**
   A. Autonomy
   B. Beneficence
   C. Non-maleficence
   D. Justice

8. **Under what circumstances is sharing a patient's health information without their explicit consent acceptable?**
   A. When discussing the case with friends outside of work
   B. In the case of a public health threat
   C. When posting about the case on social media
   D. None of the above

9. **What law ensures that all patients have the right to see and obtain a copy of their medical records?**
    A. EMTALA
    B. CLIA
    C. HIPAA
    D. FERPA

10. **What principle of medical ethics refers to doing good or acting in the best interest of patients?**
    A. Autonomy
    B. Beneficence
    C. Non-maleficence
    D. Justice

11. **What is the legal term for failing to meet the standard of care, resulting in harm to the patient?**
    A. Slander
    B. Negligence
    C. Libel
    D. Assault

12. **A healthcare professional who discloses confidential medical information could be charged with a violation of:**
    A. Autonomy
    B. Beneficence
    C. HIPAA
    D. CLIA

13. **Written defamation of character relevant to the medical field is called:**
    A. Slander
    B. Negligence
    C. Libel
    D. Assault

14. **The concept of informed consent is primarily based on which of the following ethical principles?**
    A. Autonomy
    B. Beneficence
    C. Non-maleficence
    D. Justice

15. **What action could be considered an invasion of patient privacy?**
    A. Discussing a patient's medical condition in an elevator
    B. Requiring the patient to sign a consent form before surgery
    C. Informing a patient about the side effects of a medication
    D. Listening to a patient's heart rate using a stethoscope

16. **Which ethical principle relates to fairness and equity in the delivery of healthcare?**
    A. Autonomy
    B. Beneficence
    C. Non-maleficence
    D. Justice

17. **What ethical principle requires a medical assistant to seek to do good for patients at all times?**
    A. Autonomy
    B. Beneficence
    C. Non-maleficence
    D. Justice

18. **What is considered the "double effect" in medical ethics?**
    A. When a patient experiences both positive and negative effects from a treatment
    B. When a healthcare provider's action has two effects – one beneficial and the other harmful
    C. When a healthcare provider performs two actions simultaneously
    D. When a patient needs to have two treatments at the same time

19. **Which of the following is a legally binding document that communicates a patient's wishes regarding their healthcare if they cannot communicate?**
    A. Medical history
    B. Advanced directive
    C. Consent form
    D. Health insurance policy

Communication

1. **A medical assistant should use which of the following communication techniques when speaking with a patient who has a hearing impairment?**
   - **A.** Speak loudly
   - **B.** Speak slowly and clearly
   - **C.** Use complex medical jargon
   - **D.** Avoid eye contact

2. **Which method is most effective for educating a patient about a new medication?**
   - **A.** Give the patient a printed handout and send them home
   - **B.** Explain the medication's purpose, how to take it, and side effects, and answer any questions the patient might have
   - **C.** Inform the patient to search for information online
   - **D.** Only discuss it if the patient asks

3. **What is an essential element of therapeutic communication in a healthcare setting?**
   - **A.** Providing unsolicited advice
   - **B.** Using medical jargon frequently
   - **C.** Actively listening to the patient
   - **D.** Dominating the conversation

4. **What type of communication involves body language, posture, and facial expressions?**
   - **A.** Verbal communication
   - **B.** Written communication
   - **C.** Nonverbal communication
   - **D.** Digital communication

5. **How should a medical assistant handle a situation where a patient is angry or upset?**
   - **A.** Dismiss the patient's feelings
   - **B.** Engage in an argument with the patient
   - **C.** Remain calm, listen actively, and empathize with the patient
   - **D.** Ignore the patient until they calm down

6. **Which communication skills are essential when working with a multidisciplinary healthcare team?**
   - **A.** Assertiveness
   - **B.** Passive-aggressiveness
   - **C.** Sarcasm
   - **D.** Domination

7. **In a patient-centered approach, how should a medical assistant respond if a patient does not understand medical terminology?**
   - **A.** Use more complex terminology to explain
   - **B.** Redirect the patient to a doctor
   - **C.** Re-explain using simpler, non-medical language
   - **D.** Ignore the patient's confusion

8. **When providing instructions to a patient, which strategy can help confirm the patient's understanding?**
   - **A.** Give them a written document and send them home
   - **B.** Ask them to repeat the instructions back in their own words
   - **C.** Ask them to sign a document stating they understand
   - **D.** Assume they understand if they don't ask questions

9. **Which of the following is critical to effective communication in a healthcare setting?**
    A. Disregard the feelings of the patient
    B. Use medical jargon whenever possible
    C. Empathy and understanding
    D. Frequently interrupt the patient to save time

10. **What is the primary reason for documenting patient interactions and communication in a patient's medical record?**
    A. To aid in future communication and ensure consistency of care
    B. To give the patient something to read in the waiting room
    C. To fill out the patient's file
    D. To have something to do between patient visits

11. **When speaking with a patient's emotionally distraught family member, a medical assistant should utilize what type of communication?**
    A. Confrontational communication
    B. Nonchalant communication
    C. Empathetic communication
    D. Passive communication

12. **Which strategies are essential for successful communication in a multicultural healthcare setting?**
    A. Ignoring cultural differences
    B. Enforcing stereotypes
    C. Cultural competency
    D. Exclusive language use

13. **How should a medical assistant respond to a patient who speaks quietly and rarely makes eye contact?**
    A. Ignore the behavior
    B. Demand the patient speak louder and make eye contact
    C. Adjust their communication style to match the patient's comfort level
    D. Talk about the patient with other staff members

14. **What is the importance of using plain language when communicating with patients about their health?**
    A. It prevents the medical assistant from needing to use complex medical terms
    B. It ensures that the patient understands the information being conveyed
    C. It's less time-consuming than explaining medical terms
    D. It's not essential; patients should research medical terms on their own

15. **In healthcare settings, what does active listening involve?**
    A. Only paying attention to the words spoken
    B. Dismissing non-verbal cues
    C. Listening attentively, responding appropriately, and confirming understanding
    D. Multitasking while the patient is speaking

16. **Which of the following is considered a barrier to effective communication in healthcare?**
    A. use of plain language
    B. use of medical jargon
    C. Active listening
    D. Empathy

17. **When a patient is upset, which of the following responses is the most appropriate?**
    A. "Calm down. It's not a big deal."
    B. "I understand why you might feel this way. Let's work through this together."
    C. "I'm not the person to talk to about this."
    D. Ignore the patient's feelings and continue with the routine.

18. **How should a medical assistant respond if a patient asks a question they don't know the answer to?**
        A. Guess the answer
        B. Ignore the question
        C. Admit they don't know but will find out the answer or direct the question to someone who knows
        D. Change the subject

19. **Which of the following is a non-verbal communication skill that can improve patient interaction?**
        A. Looking at the clock frequently during the conversation
        B. Not making any eye contact with the patient
        C. Maintaining an open posture
        D. Crossing your arms while speaking to the patient

Billing, Coding, and Insurance

1. **Which of the following coding systems is primarily used to report procedures and services performed by healthcare providers?**
   - **A.** ICD-10-CM
   - **B.** CPT
   - **C.** HCPCS
   - **D.** DSM-5

2. **What type of insurance plan requires patients to seek healthcare from a specific network of providers?**
   - **A.** Preferred Provider Organization (PPO)
   - **B.** Health Maintenance Organization (HMO)
   - **C.** Fee-for-Service
   - **D.** Point of Service (POS)

3. **In medical coding, what is the term for coding to the highest level of specificity?**
   - **A.** Upcoding
   - **B.** Downcoding
   - **C.** Bundling
   - **D.** Unbundling

4. **What is the primary purpose of a patient's Explanation of Benefits (EOB)?**
   - **A.** To show the details of what the insurance covered and what the patient owes
   - **B.** To detail the patient's medical history
   - **C.** To confirm the patient's appointment schedule
   - **D.** To display the patient's dietary restrictions

5. **Which document is a legal contract between the insurance company and the policyholder which outlines the coverage's costs, benefits, and terms?**
   - **A.** Superbill
   - **B.** EOB
   - **C.** Insurance policy
   - **D.** Patient's chart

6. **What is the term for the annual amount a patient must pay out-of-pocket before the insurance company begins to cover expenses?**
   - **A.** Co-pay
   - **B.** Premium
   - **C.** Deductible
   - **D.** Capitation

7. **What term refers to grouping codes together when billing for a complete procedure rather than itemizing each step?**
   - **A.** Downcoding
   - **B.** Upcoding
   - **C.** Bundling
   - **D.** Unbundling

8. **What is the process of translating descriptions of medical diagnoses and procedures into numeric or alphanumeric designations (codes)?**
   - **A.** Medical Billing
   - **B.** Medical Transcription
   - **C.** Medical Coding
   - **D.** Medical Administration

9. **According to their insurance policy, what fixed amount must a patient pay during service?**
   A. Deductible
   B. Premium
   C. Co-pay
   D. Capitation

10. **Which coding system is used to document diagnoses and clinical findings?**
    A. ICD-10-CM
    B. CPT
    C. HCPCS
    D. DSM-5

11. **What term refers to a list of charges or established allowances for specific medical services and procedures?**
    A. Superbill
    B. Fee schedule
    C. Explanation of Benefits (EOB)
    D. Insurance claim

12. **What does the abbreviation HCPCS stand for?**
    A. Healthcare Common Procedural Coding System
    B. Health Coverage and Payment Coding System
    C. Hospital Coding and Payment Classification System
    D. Health Complication and Procedure Coding System

13. **Which document contains detailed information about a patient visit, including the diagnosis, treatment provided, and the charges for services?**
    A. Insurance claim
    B. Explanation of Benefits (EOB)
    C. Superbill
    D. Fee schedule

14. **What is the term for the fraudulent practice of billing separately for procedures usually covered under a bundled code?**
    A. Downcoding
    B. Unbundling
    C. Upcoding
    D. Overcoming

15. **In healthcare, what does the term 'capitation' refer to?**
    A. The maximum limit on the amount that can be claimed from insurance
    B. A payment arrangement in which providers are paid a set amount for each enrolled person
    C. The process of confirming whether a patient's insurance is active and what services it covers
    D. The amount a patient pays out-of-pocket for services before insurance coverage begins

16. **What does the abbreviation 'EOB' stand for in the context of healthcare billing?**
    A. Estimated Overall Bill
    B. Explanation of Benefits
    C. Estimated Out-of-pocket Bill
    D. Explanation of Billing

17. **What does 'prior authorization' refer to in the context of medical services?**
    A. approval from the patient to perform the medical services
    B. approval from a healthcare provider to perform medical services
    C. Approval from an insurance company before a provider can carry out a service for a patient
    D. Approval from a medical board to carry out a specific medical service

18. **What term refers to charging a patient for the difference between the doctor's fee and the insurance provider's allowable charge?**
    A. Deductible
    B. Co-payment
    C. Balance billing
    D. Capitation

Schedule Appointments and Health Information Management

1. **What is a primary consideration when scheduling patient appointments?**
   A. The patient's insurance carrier
   B. The patient's availability
   C. The patient's marital status
   D. The patient's social status

2. **Which of the following scheduling systems assigns a specific time for each patient, spaced at regular intervals?**
   A. Wave scheduling
   B. Cluster scheduling
   C. Open booking
   D. Time-specific scheduling

3. **The process of reviewing, updating, and ensuring the accuracy, consistency, and reliability of data in health information systems is known as:**
   A. Data scrubbing
   B. Data reconciliation
   C. Data mapping
   D. Data validation

4. **What is the primary purpose of a patient's health record?**
   A. To track billing and insurance information
   B. To provide a complete and accurate account of the patient's medical history
   C. To record patient-staff communication
   D. To promote the practice on social media

5. **The act of scheduling two patients to see the doctor at the same time is known as:**
   A. Double booking
   B. Cluster scheduling
   C. Open booking
   D. Wave scheduling

6. **What does the term 'interoperability' refer to in health information management?**
   A. The ability of health information systems to work within and across organizational boundaries
   B. The ability to prevent unauthorized access to patient records
   C. The ability to delete patient records
   D. The ability to copy patient records

7. **Which of the following is a type of scheduling where multiple patients are given the same appointment time and are seen in the order they arrive?**
   A. Cluster scheduling
   B. Wave scheduling
   C. Open booking
   D. Time-specific scheduling

8. **Which law in the United States protects the privacy of a patient's personal health information?**
   A. The Affordable Care Act
   B. The Health Insurance Portability and Accountability Act (HIPAA)
   C. The Medicare Access and CHIP Reauthorization Act
   D. The Americans with Disabilities Act

9. **In health information management, the term 'data integrity refers to:**
   A. The completeness, accuracy, and reliability of data during collection, processing, storage, and distribution
   B. The quantity of data collected
   C. The types of data collected
   D. The speed of data collection

10. **What is the most efficient way to handle a patient who frequently misses scheduled appointments?**
    A. Schedule them for the last appointment of the day
    B. Double book their appointment slot
    C. Require a deposit for booking an appointment
    D. Discuss the importance of appointments and adherence to the schedule

11. **What scheduling system is designed to reduce waiting times and prevent gaps in a provider's schedule by dividing each hour into 10- to 20-minute slots and scheduling two to four patients every half hour?**
    A. Wave scheduling
    B. Double booking
    C. Cluster scheduling
    D. Open booking

12. **Which of the following is a software application used to store and manage patients' health information?**
    A. Electronic Health Records (EHR)
    B. Healthcare Data Warehouse
    C. Patient Management System
    D. Integrated Delivery System

13. **A patient who the provider has not seen within the past three years would be considered as a(n):**
    A. Established patient
    B. New patient
    C. Outpatient
    D. Inpatient

14. **What is the process of ensuring a patient's appointment is scheduled at a time when any necessary preceding steps (like fasting or taking medications) can occur?**
    A. Buffering
    B. Preauthorization
    C. Previsit planning
    D. Staggering

15. **Which term refers to the ability to gain access to and use health information when and where it is needed?**
    A. Interoperability
    B. Data accessibility
    C. Information governance
    D. Data integrity

16. **In health information management, a 'Master Patient Index (MPI)' is:**
    A. A list of all health problems and diagnoses for a patient
    B. A list of all patients who have ever been treated in a facility
    C. A system used to identify specific treatments given to a patient
    D. A system used to track patient appointments and visits

Which type of appointment scheduling allows for continuity of care but may have periods of downtime for the physician?

      A. Wave scheduling

      B. Stream scheduling

      C. Cluster scheduling

      D. Double booking

17. **What term describes the transfer of electronic health information from one healthcare system to another and its use in a meaningful way?**

      A. Data integration

      B. Information governance

      C. Interoperability

      D. Data mapping

Answer Key

Clinical Workflow: Patient Intake and Discharge

1. Correct answer: **C.** Verify patient's identity. The patient's identity should be confirmed before action as a standard safety measure.
2. Correct answer: **D.** All of the above. All this information is critical for creating a comprehensive patient profile.
3. Correct answer: **C.** Prescribing medications. CMAs typically don't have the authority to prescribe drugs; that's the physician's responsibility.
4. Correct answer: **D.** All of the above. All these factors are essential to ensure the follow-up appointment is effective and timely.
5. Correct answer: **C.** Informed Consent form. This document ensures that the patient understands and consents to the proposed treatment plan.
6. Correct answer: **C.** Call the insurance company to verify coverage. It's essential to confirm insurance details before proceeding.
7. Correct answer: **C.** During the first visit. Patients need to understand their privacy rights as early as possible.
8. Correct answer: **C.** The physician. While a CMA assists in implementing the care plan, the physician is primarily responsible for its development.
9. Correct answer: **B.** Making sure the patient understands their care plan. Patient understanding is crucial to ensure adherence to the care plan.
10. Correct answer: **C.** After the patient's appointment. This allows for a comprehensive overview of the selection and the next steps for the patient's care.
11. Correct answer: **D.** All of the above. These are standard vital signs a CMA should check during patient intake.
12. Correct answer: **B.** Sending a complete patient health record to the new provider. It's essential for continuity of care that the new provider has access to the patient's health information.
13. Correct answer: **B.** False. CMAs can provide general health information but should not offer medical advice as it's outside their scope of practice.
14. Correct answer: **C.** Reach the patient to inquire about their absence. It's essential to understand why the patient missed the appointment before deciding on the next steps.
15. Correct answer: **B.** How to administer the medication. They must understand how to take their prescribed medication correctly for patient safety.
16. Correct answer: **B.** The minor's guardian or parent. Generally, a parent or legal guardian must consent to medical procedures involving children.
17. Correct answer: **B.** Administer first aid and call for emergency medical services. CMAs are trained to provide first aid and should call for emergency medical assistance when necessary.
18. Correct answer: **A.** Patient Health Information. PHI refers to any information in a medical record that can be used to identify an individual.
19. Correct answer: **D.** Proceed with the appointment, but inform the patient that it may need to be cut short. This option maintains the patient's care but also respects the schedule of other patients.
20. Correct answer: **B.** The CM**A.** The CMA often takes on this role, although the physician may also be involved depending on the case's complexity.
21. Correct answer: **C.** To obtain the patient's medical history and demographic information. An intake form serves as a basis for patient profiling and treatment planning.
22. Correct answer: **C.** Explain again using simpler terms or provide additional resources. CMAs must ensure patients understand their care instructions upon discharge.
23. Correct answer: **C.** The patient's medical necessity. While other factors matter, the patient's health needs should always be the primary consideration.

24. Correct answer: **A.** Ask the patient to verify their name and date of birth. This method is widely used, simple, and efficient in confirming patient identity.

25. Correct answer: **B.** Document the refusal in the patient's medical recor**D.** The patient has the right to refuse treatment, and this decision should be appropriately documented.

26. Correct answer: **C.** Both verbal and written instructions. This ensures the patient fully understands their care plan and can reference the instructions later.

27. Correct answer: **C.** Discuss the discrepancy with the patient for clarification. It's essential to have accurate patient information for effective healthcare delivery.

Safety and Infection Control

1. Correct answer: **A.** OSH**A.** The Occupational Safety and Health Administration (OSHA) enforces regulations to protect healthcare workers.
2. Correct answer: **C.** Placing it in a designated, clearly marked container. This is standard protocol to ensure safety and minimize the risk of infection.
3. Correct answer: **C.** Absence of pathogens. Asepsis refers to the state of being free from disease-causing microorganisms.
4. Correct answer: **A.** Using gloves when touching blood, body fluids, secretions, and excretions. This is a universal standard precaution to prevent the spread of infections.
5. Correct answer: **B.** When dealing with a patient with an airborne disease like T**B.** N95 masks provide respiratory protection against airborne infections.
6. Correct answer: **B.** To protect the healthcare worker from potential exposure to infectious materials. PPE serves to protect the wearer from various health and safety hazards.
7. Correct answer: **C.** Notify your supervisor or responsible personnel. They can assess the situation and determine the appropriate course of action.
8. Correct answer: **B.** In a designated sharps container. This is to prevent needlestick injuries and possible spread of infection.
9. Correct answer: **C.** Hand hygiene. While other precautions are essential, hand hygiene is considered the most critical method to prevent the spread of germs.
10. Correct answer: **B.** Wash the area with soap and water. Afterward, they should report the incident to their supervisor and follow their facility's protocol for such injuries.
11. Correct answer: **A.** Gown, mask/respirator, goggles/face shield, gloves. This is the standard sequence the Centers for Disease Control and Prevention (CDC) recommends.
12. Correct answer: **A.** Only sterilized equipment and supplies must be used. This principle ensures that the operating environment is free from microorganisms.
13. Correct answer: **C.** CO2 extinguisher. Using a CO2 extinguisher on an electrical fire is safer as it doesn't leave a residue that can harm the equipment.
14. Correct answer: **A.** Communicable. These diseases can be transmitted directly or indirectly from one person to another.
15. Correct answer: **C.** Tuberculosis. While it's a severe infectious disease, tuberculosis is primarily a respiratory pathogen, not bloodborne.
16. Correct answer: **C.** Airborne precautions. These diseases are transmitted through tiny droplets that can linger in the air, requiring unique airborne isolation rooms.
17. Correct answer: **C.** Before and after every patient interaction, after touching potentially contaminated surfaces, and before putting on and after removing PPE. Frequent hand hygiene is the best defense against spreading infections.
18. Correct answer: **B.** Material Safety Data Sheet. It provides detailed information about a specific hazardous substance, including how to handle, store, and dispose of it safely.
19. Correct answer: **B.** Rinse the eye with water or saline for at least 15 minutes. Then, report the incident to a supervisor and seek medical attention if necessary.
20. Correct answer: **B.** To provide an extra layer of protection against leaks or tears. This practice adds a level of safety for those handling the waste.
21. Correct answer: **D.** Autoclaving effectively cleans instruments but does not sterilize them. This statement is false. Autoclaving is a sterilization process, not merely a cleaning process.
22. Correct answer: **C.** Infectious waste. Red bags or containers are typically used for infectious waste, including blood, body fluids, and other potentially infectious material.
23. Correct answer: **B.** To provide important information about potential hazards and safety precautions for handling, storing, and transporting chemicals. The SDS is a crucial reference for safe chemical management.
24. Correct answer: **B.** Immediately wash the exposed area with soap and water. Quick action is crucial in reducing the risk of infection.
25. Correct answer: **B.** Personal Protective Equipment. PPE is worn to minimize exposure to hazards and includes gloves, masks, gowns, and eyewear.
26. Correct answer: **A.** Hepatitis A and **B.** Currently, vaccines are available to prevent Hepatitis A and B, but not C, D, or E.

27. Correct answer: **D.** Spray in a circular motion. The proper method is to spray back and forth in a controlled manner, not in a circular motion.

Procedures/Examinations

1. Correct answer: **B.** The second intercostal space is at the left sternal border. This location is known as the aortic area, where sounds from the aortic valve are best heard.
2. Correct answer: **B.** Visual acuity. The Snellen Test is a standard eye test used to determine a patient's visual acuity or clarity of vision.
3. Correct answer: **A.** Otoscopic examination. While a neurological exam may also be indicated, vertigo is often related to issues in the inner ear which can be examined using an otoscope.
4. Correct answer: **B.** Gallbladder disease. Murphy's sign is a clinical maneuver during which the patient is asked to take a deep breath while the doctor presses on the right upper quadrant of the abdomen.
5. Correct answer: **C.** Sims'. The Sims' position, with the patient lying on their left side, is commonly used for rectal and vaginal examinations.
6. Correct answer: **C.** After the last tube has been filled and the needle is withdrawn. This is to minimize any tissue damage under the tourniquet and avoid hemoconcentration.
7. Correct answer: **B.** Non-absorbable sutures. These sutures are solid and durable, making them suitable for high-tension areas where the suture needs to remain in place for extended periods.
8. Correct answer: **D.** To monitor heart rhythms. An ECG measures the electrical activity of the heart to identify any irregularities.
9. Correct answer: **C.** Cervix. A Pap smear involves collecting cells from the cervix to screen for cervical cancer.
10. Correct answer: **B.** Endoscopy. This procedure allows for the visual examination of a body cavity or organ.
11. Correct answer: **A.** Right upper quadrant. The liver is located in the right upper quadrant of the abdomen.
12. Correct answer: **C.** Palpation. This technique involves the healthcare provider using their hands to feel the body.
13. Correct answer: **B.** Prone. In the prone position, the patient lies on their stomach, which allows the healthcare provider to examine the back of the chest best.
14. Correct answer: **C.** The back of the throat. This is where the bacteria causing strep throat are most likely found.
15. Correct answer: **A.** Inner ear dysfunction. The Romberg test assesses balance and can indicate problems with the inner ear or sensory system.
16. Correct answer: **B.** To monitor heart rhythm continuously over 24 hours. This provides a more comprehensive view of heart activity than a single ECG.
17. Correct answer: **C.** Median cubital vein. This vein, located in the antecubital fossa, is typically easy to identify and is relatively large.
18. Correct answer: **D.** All of the above. These are all appropriate sites for intramuscular injection, but the choice depends on various factors, including medication volume and patient age, size, and condition.
19. Correct answer: **D.** Magnetic resonance imaging (MRI). MRI scans provide detailed images of soft tissues, organs, and other structures within the body.
20. Correct answer: **B.** Pulse oximeter. A pulse oximeter is a non-invasive device that estimates oxygen saturation in a patient's blood.
21. Correct answer: **A.** McBurney's point tenderness. This is a standard examination technique in which pressure is applied to the lower right quadrant of the abdomen (McBurney's point), where the appendix is typically located.
22. Correct answer: **C.** MRI. Magnetic resonance imaging is especially suited for detailed imaging of soft tissues, including ligaments, muscles, and tendons.
23. Correct answer: **B.** Creatinine. The kidneys filter this waste product of muscle metabolism, which is a standard indicator of kidney function.
24. Correct answer: **A.** Supine. With the patient lying flat, the jugular veins will be at the same level as the heart, facilitating the assessment of jugular venous pressure.
25. Correct answer: **B.** To visualize the bronchi and diagnose lung conditions. A bronchoscopy involves inserting a bronchoscope into the patient's airways to observe the bronchi and lungs.

26. Correct answer: **D.** Both A and **C.** In a glucose tolerance test, blood samples are typically taken before the trial begins (fasting blood glucose) and then at regular intervals after the patient drinks a glucose solution.
27. Correct answer: **C.** Holter monitor. A Holter monitor records the heart's activity continuously for 24 hours, providing a more detailed picture of heart function than a single ECG.
28. Correct answer: **B.** To evaluate lung function. Spirometry measures the volume and speed of breaths, helping diagnose conditions such as asthma and COPD.
29. Correct answer: **D.** X-ray. X-rays are beneficial for visualizing bones and identifying any fractures or abnormalities.

Pharmacology

1. Correct answer: **A.** Diuretics. These drugs work by causing the kidneys to remove more sodium and water from the body, which helps to relax the blood vessel walls and lower blood pressure.
2. Correct answer: **B.** Relieve pain. Opioids are drugs known for their potent analgesic (pain-relieving) effects.
3. Correct answer: **B.** Amoxicillin. This antibiotic medication is commonly used to treat various bacterial infections.
4. Correct answer: **B.** To increase urine output. Diuretics are often called 'water pills' because they help remove excess water from the body through increased urine production.
5. Correct answer: **C.** Intravenous. This route allows the medication to be delivered directly into the bloodstream, providing the fastest onset of action.
6. Correct answer: **A.** Anaphylaxis. This is a severe, systemic allergic reaction that requires immediate medical attention.
7. Correct answer: **C.** Metformin. This is a standard first-line treatment for type 2 diabetes.
8. Correct answer: **A.** Benzodiazepines. These medications are frequently used to treat anxiety and panic disorders.
9. Correct answer: **B.** Prevent blood clot formation. Anticoagulants, or "blood thinners," slow down the body's process of forming clots.
10. Correct answer: **A.** Ibuprofen. It is an NSAID commonly used to relieve pain, reduce inflammation, and lower fever.
11. Correct answer: **B.** Fluoxetine. It is a selective serotonin reuptake inhibitor (SSRI) frequently used to treat depression.
12. Correct answer: **A.** Naloxone. It can rapidly reverse an opioid overdose by binding to opioid receptors, blocking the effects of other opioids.
13. Correct answer: **B.** Zidovudine. This antiretroviral medication is used to prevent and treat HIV/AIDS.
14. Correct answer: **C.** Antiarrhythmics. They work by suppressing abnormal rhythms of the heart (arrhythmias).
15. Correct answer: **C.** NSAIDs. Long-term use of NSAIDs can irritate the stomach lining and increase the risk of ulcers.
16. Correct answer: **B.** Albuterol. It's a bronchodilator that relaxes muscles in the airways and increases airflow to the lungs.
17. Correct answer: **C.** Statins. They work by reducing levels of bad cholesterol in the blood.
18. Correct answer: **C.** Carbamazepine. This anticonvulsant medication is frequently used to control seizures.
19. Correct answer: **D.** Losartan. This angiotensin II receptor antagonist can treat high blood pressure and help treat BPH.
20. Correct answer: **A.** To prevent or reduce nausea and vomiting. Antiemetic drugs work by blocking the signals to the part of the brain that triggers nausea and vomiting.
21. Correct answer: **C.** Levothyroxine. It's a synthetic form of thyroxine, the hormone produced by the thyroid gland.
22. Correct answer: **B.** Beta-blockers. They can decrease intraocular fluid production and lower elevated intraocular pressure.
23. Correct answer: **A.** Diphenhydramine. This antihistamine is often used to treat symptoms of allergies, including sneezing, runny nose, itching, and watery eyes.

Legal and Ethical Issues

1. Correct answer: **A.** HIPAA. The Health Insurance Portability and Accountability Act (HIPAA) requires the confidentiality and secure handling of protected health information.
2. Correct answer: **C.** Non-maleficence. It is the principle of "not harm" and is a fundamental precept in healthcare.
3. Correct answer: **B.** Leaving a patient's medical records open in public. This would be an example of a breach of confidentiality as it could expose the patient's protected health information.
4. Correct answer: **A.** Autonomy. This principle supports the right of the patient to have control over their healthcare decisions.
5. Correct answer: **A.** EMTALA. The Emergency Medical Treatment and Labor Act (EMTALA) requires that emergency care be provided regardless of a patient's ability to pay.
6. Correct answer: **C.** Report it to a supervisor or the practice's compliance officer. Any suspicions of illegal or unethical behavior should be reported to the appropriate authority in the organization.
7. Correct answer: **D.** Justice. This principle involves fairness and equality in the distribution of resources and the application of healthcare treatment.
8. Correct answer: **B.** In the case of a public health threat. Under certain circumstances, such as public health emergencies, healthcare providers may be required to report certain information to public health departments or other authorities.
9. Correct answer: **C.** HIPAA. The Health Insurance Portability and Accountability Act (HIPAA) gives patients the right to access and obtain a copy of their health information.
10. Correct answer: **B.** Beneficence. This principle refers to the obligation to act in the patient's best interests and to promote good over harm.
11. Correct answer: **B.** Negligence. Negligence occurs when a healthcare professional fails to provide the standard of care, harming the patient.
12. Correct answer: **C.** HIPAA. The Health Insurance Portability and Accountability Act (HIPAA) protects patient confidentiality.
13. Correct answer: **C.** Libel. Written defamatory statements in the medical field, such as false information in a patient's chart, can be considered libel.
14. Correct answer: **A.** Autonomy. Informed consent reflects the patient's right to make decisions about their healthcare.
15. Correct answer: **A.** Discussing a patient's medical condition in an elevator. Patient privacy must always be respected, and discussions about their condition should only occur in a secure, private location.
16. Correct answer: **D.** Justice. Justice refers to fairness and equity in healthcare, ensuring that all patients receive the same standard of care regardless of their circumstances.
17. Correct answer: **B.** Beneficence. The principle of beneficence directs healthcare providers to do good for the benefit of others.
18. Correct answer: **B.** When a healthcare provider's action has two beneficial and harmful effects, this often arises in palliative care cases, where pain relief may also hasten death.
19. Correct answer: **B.** Advanced directive. Advanced directives, such as living wills or durable power of attorney for healthcare, specify a patient's preferences for treatment if they become incapacitated.

Communication

1. Correct answer: **B.** Speak slowly and clearly. Clear, slow speech is essential when communicating with deaf and hard-of-hearing patients.
2. Correct answer: **B.** Explain the medication's purpose, how to take it, and side effects, and answer any questions the patient might have. This ensures the patient understands the medication's role in treatment and how to use it properly.
3. Correct answer: **C.** Actively listening to the patient. This ensures the patient feels heard and their concerns are being addressed.
4. Correct answer: **C.** Nonverbal communication. Nonverbal cues often convey meaning beyond spoken words.
5. Correct answer: **C.** Remain calm, listen actively, and empathize with the patient. This approach helps to diffuse tension and promote a more effective dialogue.
6. Correct answer: **A.** Assertiveness. Communicating needs, ideas, or concerns respectfully and confidently within a healthcare team is crucial.
7. Correct answer: **C.** Re-explain using more straightforward, non-medical language. This approach ensures that the patient understands their health condition and care instructions.
8. Correct answer: **B.** Ask them to repeat the instructions in their own words. This method, known as "teach-back," can confirm patient comprehension.
9. Correct answer: **C.** Empathy and understanding. Effective communication involves understanding the patient's perspective and responding with empathy.
10. Correct answer: **A.** To aid in future communication and ensure consistency of care. Documentation supports information continuity and enhances patient care.
11. Correct answer: **C.** Empathetic communication. Empathy allows the medical assistant to understand and share the family member's feelings, facilitating a supportive conversation.
12. Correct answer: **C.** Cultural competency. Understanding, respecting, and acknowledging cultural differences can significantly improve communication in a multicultural healthcare setting.
13. Correct answer: **C.** Adjust their communication style to match the patient's comfort level. Respectful adjustment can create a more comfortable environment for the patient.
14. Correct answer: **B.** It ensures that the patient understands the information being conveyed. The primary goal of healthcare communication is the patient's understanding.
15. Correct answer: **C.** Listening attentively, responding appropriately, and confirming understanding. Active listening is a critical component of effective communication.
16. Correct answer: **B.** Use of medical jargon. Using complex medical terms that a patient doesn't understand can prevent effective communication.
17. Correct answer: **B.** "I understand why you might feel this way. Let's work through this together." This empathetic response validates the patient's feelings and provides reassurance.
18. Correct answer: **C.** Admit they don't know but will find the answer or direct the question to someone who knows. Honesty is crucial in healthcare. The assistant should always guess or provide correct information.
19. Correct answer: **C.** Maintaining an open posture. This non-verbal cue suggests you're engaged, honest, and attentive.

Billing, Coding, and Insurance

1. Correct answer: **B.** CPT (Current Procedural Terminology). The CPT coding system reports medical, surgical, and diagnostic procedures and services.
2. Correct answer: **B.** Health Maintenance Organization (HMO). HMO plans generally require patients to select a primary care physician (PCP) within the network.
3. Correct answer: **A.** Upcoding. Upcoding refers to using a billing code that provides a higher reimbursement rate for the service rendered.
4. Correct answer: **A.** To show the details of what the insurance covers and what the patient owes. The EOB is a statement from the insurance company explaining what services were paid, denied, or reduced in payment.
5. Correct answer: **C.** Insurance policy. This document outlines the full details of an insurance agreement.
6. Correct answer: **C.** Deductible. A deductible is the amount a patient must pay for covered services before the insurance starts to pay.
7. Correct answer: **C.** Bundling. Bundling refers to grouping codes to reflect the procedure rather than billing separately for each process step.
8. Correct answer: **C.** Medical Coding. Medical Coding involves translating patients' case histories into applicable medical codes.
9. Correct answer: **C.** Co-pay. A co-pay is a predetermined rate a patient pays for healthcare services at the time of care.
10. Correct answer: **A.** ICD-10-CM. International Classification of Diseases, Tenth Revision, Clinical Modification (ICD-10-CM) is a system healthcare providers use to classify and code diagnoses and symptoms.
11. Correct answer: **B.** Fee schedule. A fee schedule is a list of the amounts that are allowed to be billed for a particular medical service.
12. Correct answer: **A.** Healthcare Common Procedural Coding System. HCPCS reports medical procedures and equipment to Medicare and other health insurers.
13. Correct answer: **C.** Superbill. A superbill includes all information about a patient visit needed to prepare an insurance claim.
14. Correct answer: **B.** Unbundling. Unbundling refers to separating a group of procedures to increase billing.
15. Correct answer: **B.** A payment arrangement in which providers are paid a set amount for each enrolled person. Capitation is a payment model that pays providers a set amount for each enrolled person assigned to them per period, whether or not that person seeks care.
16. Correct answer: **B.** Explanation of Benefits. An EOB is a document sent by an insurance company to a patient explaining what was covered for a medical service and how much they must pay the provider directly if anything.
17. Correct answer: **C.** An insurance company approves before a provider can carry out a service for a patient. Prior authorization requires a healthcare provider to obtain approval from the health insurance plan to prescribe a specific medication, procedure, or service.
18. Correct answer: **C.** Balance billing. Balance billing happens when providers bill patients for the difference between the amount they charge and the amount the insurance pays.

Schedule Appointments and Health Information Management

1. Correct answer: **B.** The patient's availability. While all factors may have some importance, the patient's schedule is typically the primary factor considered when setting appointments.
2. Correct answer: **D.** Time-specific scheduling. This method assigns a specific time slot to each patient during the day.
3. Correct answer: **A.** Data scrubbing. It's the process of cleaning and harmonizing the data.
4. Correct answer: **B.** To provide a complete and accurate account of the patient's medical history. It's essential for coordinating care.
5. Correct answer: **A.** Double booking. This is when two patients are given the same appointment slot with the same provider.
6. Correct answer: **A.** The ability of health information systems to work within and across organizational boundaries. Interoperability allows for the sharing and using patient information across different health information systems.
7. Correct answer: **C.** Open booking. This system allows for flexibility but may also lead to long wait times if many patients arrive simultaneously.
8. Correct answer: **B.** The Health Insurance Portability and Accountability Act (HIPAA). This law sets the standard for protecting sensitive patient data.
9. Correct answer: **A.** The completeness, accuracy, and reliability of data during collection, processing, storage, and distribution. Data integrity is crucial for maintaining trust in the data and the systems that store and process such data.
10. Correct answer: **D.** Discuss the importance of appointments and adherence to the schedule. Open communication is always a beneficial approach.
11. Correct answer: **A.** Wave scheduling. This system helps maintain a steady flow of patients throughout the day.
12. Correct answer: **A.** Electronic Health Records (EHR). EHRs are real-time, patient-centered records that provide instant and secure information to authorized users.
13. Correct answer: **B.** New patient. According to most healthcare providers and insurance companies, a patient is considered "new" if they haven't been seen by the provider or a provider of the same specialty within the same practice for three years.
14. Correct answer: **C.** Previsit planning. It ensures that any necessary preparations are accounted for when scheduling an appointment.
15. Correct answer: **B.** Data accessibility. It's crucial to ensure that healthcare providers can access the data they need to provide adequate care.
16. Correct answer: **B.** A list of all patients who have ever been treated in a facility. The MPI helps in keeping track of all the patients.
17. Correct answer: **B.** Stream scheduling. Stream scheduling, or time-specific scheduling, allows for one-on-one interaction between the physician and the patient but can lead to downtime if patients cancel or are no-shows.
18. Correct answer: **C.** Interoperability. This is a critical component of effective health information management, as it allows for information to be shared and used across multiple systems.

MASTERING THE CMA EXAM: PROVEN TIPS AND TECHNIQUES

The path toward becoming a Certified Medical Assistant (CMA) is an honorable endeavor that proves the dedication to professionalism in medical assisting. However, the CMA exam is a doorway to this prestigious title, and it tests your clinical and administrative skills, among many other responsibilities. This list of established approaches can enable you to study effectively for the test.

Understand the Exam Structure
Indeed, before we plunge into demystifying study materials' thorny issues, we must shed light on the CMA Examination's construct. Become familiar with the format that usually consists of multiple-choice questions on selected areas relevant to medical assisting. Understanding the design can eliminate demystification and modify your study process.

Create a Study Plan
Your study plan for the same must be structured. Some of the topics you need to cover, then set aside time for every case based on the amount in your exam and how good you are at that. Your schedule with such short breaks efficiently increases your retention and avoids burnout.

Utilize Official Study Materials
Get guides and aids that feature from AAMA, the certified medical assistant exam. It has tailored resources designed according to the exam content outline. Hence, you will study what is relevant.

Join Study Groups
It is generally accepted that two heads are better than one, and preparing for an exam refers to this term. A study group will also provide moral support, diverse, challenging insights, and discuss all topics repeatedly, creating reinforcement of learning.

Incorporate Diverse Learning Methods
Everyone learns differently. The difference in their preferred learning style is that some know better using visual means, such as charts and videos, while others like reading or practicing. Use various methods to discover the most convenient for you and make the study routine enjoyable.

Practice, Practice, Practice
Practice Tests Are Not Negotiable. They make you confident with exam modality and time stress. In addition, regular practice will show you what areas need more study.

Understand Common Medical Terminology
Understanding medical terminology is of extreme importance while working as a medical assistant. Ensure you know basic medical terminology, abbreviations, and symbols used in health care.

Master Administrative Skills
This test covers administrative procedures—everything from scheduling appointments to filing insurance. Familiarize yourself with the latest practice in these areas.

Brush Up on Clinical Knowledge
The exam consists of a significant chunk of clinical tasks. Procedures for Reviewing the Essentials of Taking Vital Signs, Preparing Patients for Examination, and Understanding Basic Pharmacology.

Staying Abreast with Law and Ethics.
The CMA exam mandates that the two should be learned. Stay updated on the issues of patient privacy laws, for example, HIPAA, informed consent, and medical records.

Time Management during the Exam
Maintain a consistent rate during the exam. Take time for each question, especially on the challenging questions. Sometimes, you need to mark questions for future clarification if time allows.

Healthy Lifestyle Choices
A sound mind dwells in a healthy body. Sleep well, eat properly, and observe routine exercise during your preparations. Cognitive function and concentration can also be improved by reducing stress with the help of relaxation techniques or training.

Seek Feedback
Feel free to ask for assistance if you experience difficulties in a particular situation—contact instructors, colleagues, or professionals in the discipline who can clarify points that need to be understood.

Stay Positive and Confident
Finally, one has to be positive. When you prepare well, confidence will come; trust yourself that you have worked hard. Remember that your aim is to study for exams and start an exciting journey of becoming a certified medical assistant.

Finally, to prepare for the CMA exam is a long run. This is about thoughtful, consistent study in tandem with familiarizing yourself with your learning style. Referring to these tips will ensure that you complete your study material fast, be well-prepared for the examination, and be confident in becoming a CMA.

It is difficult for the best of students to tame their anxieties on exam day. Knowing how to manage this stress is just as important as knowing the material. On the spectrum, we discuss a range of tactics to stay calm and maximize performance on the CMA exam.

Navigating Exam Day: Stress Management and Effective Test-Taking Strategies

Before the Exam
- **Preparation Is Key:** Sleep well, have a good breakfast, and be prepared to create a pleasant atmosphere. Come to the testing center earlier, as well.
- **Visualize Success:** Take a few minutes and imagine yourself having a successful experience in the exam. Such positive mental rehearsal can elevate a person's confidence and minimize anxiety.
- **Breathing Techniques:** Use deep breathing exercises if nerves begin to bring on the fraying. The relaxation response can be activated by taking slow, deliberate breaths that reduce the heart rate and relax the mind.
- **Stretch and Move:** A little physical activity or stretching before entering the exam room exposes the brain to more oxygen and blood that can help clarify our minds and calm us down.

During the Exam
- **Read Carefully:** Read each question thoroughly. Be careful to avoid this common pitfall of misunderstanding the question, so get sure of what is asked before you start to answer.
- **Strategic Approach:** Address your vital questions to begin with. It can give you the confidence to get all your easy points out of the way before moving on to more complex questions.
- **Time Management:** Watch the clock, but not by it. Develop a rhythm that makes you take enough time on each question without hurrying.
- **Answer Selection:** If you are unsure of an answer, eliminate the possible incorrect answers and make a good guess from those left. On some occasions, even subsequent questions can give clues.
- **Pace Yourself: Don't rush.** Take time to think about each answer and beat the clock on any question. If you cannot solve it, then highlight it and move forward at that time. When there is a vacant period processed, return to the question again.

- **Change Answers Judiciously:** Change answers only if they give you a positive reason to believe your first answer was incorrect. You often realize your first choice is suitable if you read the question correctly.
- **Mind Mapping:** Create a brief mind map or list for complex questions & see the problem visually first, then pick an answer.
- **Stay Hydrated:** Finally, dehydration may result in fatigue and declining cognitive ability. If possible, drink or wet lips in the examination to remain doused with water.

Managing Stress during the Exam

- **Stay Present:** If you realize your mind is wandering to the likely results of the exam, then gently bring back your focus on this particular question. Increasing concentration through engaging in the "here and now."
- **Positive Affirmations:** Replace with positive self–directed thoughts. Remember how hard you worked and what you know.
- **Break down the Exam:** Think of the exam as made up of many small parts; you can handle each piece separately. This can help you to take the scare out of the exam question so that you may concentrate on what needs to be done.
- **Body Scan Relaxation:** Take a moment and do a quick body scan for tension, especially in your shoulders, neck, or jaw, and physically relax tight muscles.
- **Focus on Effort, Not Outcome:** You can only control the effort you put into every question but not necessarily the outcome. Try to focus on providing your best response to every question.

After the Exam
- **Debrief Calmly:** It is expected to analyze your performance, but try not to debrief right away with peers as it can often increase anxiety. Allow yourself time to decompress.
- **Reward Yourself:** Do something fun after the exam. Such positivity you will feel is rewarding and serves as a relief to stress after that maddening struggle.
- **Reflect:** When relaxed, take the tally of all things that went well and those you should improve. This will be very useful in your following exams and the future of your career.

Integrating such strategies into your exam-day rituals can help address the issue of stress and increase your ability to show how much you know. However, you must remember that the CMA exam is just a part of the journey and not an achievement in-complete. The secrets to success are your preparation, self-care, and becoming an SAT-like test-taking machine.

QUESTIONS AND ANSWERS

Question: Why is confidentiality important in Medical Law and Ethics?
Answer: The first problem in medical law and ethics is confidentiality, where healthcare providers should protect patient's information. It also gives patients confidence in their healthcare providers such that they can trust them with sensitive information without fear of it falling into the wrong hands. Confidentiality breaches may be illegal and unethical and lead to a deterioration in the doctor-patient relationship.

Question: Explain PHI AND PHI in health care.
Answer: Protected Health Information (PHI): any health information regarding a patient or individual, past, present, and future, that could be used to identify the given individual. One should realize that PHI is provided importance by the Health Insurance Portability and Accountability Act (HIPAA). Compliance with the HIPAA rule protects PHI and patient privacy and data from intrusion.

Question: What law aims to safeguard patient information privacy and control access to health records?
Answer: The Health Insurance Portability and Accountability Act (HIPAA) is responsible for ensuring that patients' privacy is upheld and controlling access to health records. This is important because while HIPAA covers privacy and security standards, PHI/HIPAA regulates the sharing of a client's health information.

Question: Why Program Goals for OSHA Behavior?
Answer: The Occupational Safety and Health Administration (OSHA) is established to ensure the safety of the workplace as well as protect workers from hazards. OSHA regulations in healthcare refer to infection control and hazardous materials associated with the healthcare environment.

Question: Explain Autonomy in medical ethics.
Answer: Autonomy in medical ethics is defined as the power of a patient to choose their healthcare, such as agreeing to or rejecting treatment. Therefore, accepting a patient's choices and decisions within reason, even though they may contradict the provider's recommendations, will be the central point of care unless a patient can be classified as unreasonable.

Question: What is an EMR, and what can it do for healthcare?
Answer: An EMR is an individual's computerized medical chart. This assists health care in keeping records well, data accessibility reduces errors and enhances coordination with health care providers. Through this, the EMRs help ensure that patient's information is up to date and accurate.

Question: What is a crucial advantage of stream scheduling in a medical setting?
Answer: Stream scheduling is an appointment system that schedules patients for set periods throughout the day. Third, it helps reduce patient waiting time, optimizing healthcare providers' utilization. It enhances patient satisfaction and maximizes clinic operations.

Question: What matters in a patient scheduling system?
Answer: In managing a patient's appointment schedule, it is essential to keep in mind the medical needs of the patient, time constraints, and provider availability. Scheduling should be done with first preference given to urgent cases. Secondly, it helps make appointments for a patient and store preferences so that overbooked and missed appointments are controlled.

Question: How often do you need to practice hand hygiene in a medical setting?
Answer: To this end, hand hygiene must be done routinely in a healthcare context, such as before and after every patient contact, after touching any probably contaminated surface, and when the hands are dirty. Observing hand hygiene is an essential action towards controlling infections in healthcare environments.

Question: What does PPE mean in medical terms?
Answer: The term refers to "Personal Protective Equipment," including, for example, gloves, masks, gowns, and goggles that a healthcare giver employs to protect himself and patients against any infection.

Question: Why is patient consent relevant in doing any procedure?
Answer: Obtaining patient consent is essential before performing any medical procedure to allow for Autonomy by the patients and to enable them to make informed decisions regarding their health. This is a legal and ethical protection from liability to the health care providers. Informed consent consists of an extensive briefing about the conduct of a procedure, potential hazards, advantages, and substitutions.

Question: What does medical coding do for healthcare?
Answer: This process of translating healthcare services and diagnoses into alphanumeric codes is called medical coding. It is crucial in healthcare since it supports accurate billing, the enhancement of insurance claims, and the availability of research data, which is critical for healthcare quality improvement. The financial viability of healthcare facilities and the accuracy of medical records depend on proper medical coding.

Question: Explain Certified Medical Assistant and Patient Education—analysis of the Role.
Answer: Patient education is often essential for Certified Medical Assistants (CMAs). They educate patients on their medical conditions, treatment plans, drugs, and what to do to live with their medical condition. Educating the patients is a knowledge sharing that enables them to make informed choices related to their health care, thus improving the quality of recovery.

Question: What is the significance of maintaining accurate patient records?
Answer: Quality healthcare is dependent on maintaining accurate patient records. Continuity of care is assured, and a buyer can make an informed decision supporting legal documentation and improved patient safety. Proper record keeping also facilitates good communication among team members in healthcare.

Question: Why is Insurance Verification Essential for Patients?
Answer: Insurance coverage is essential to ensure that the patient and healthcare facility do not face any financial issues. This aids the patients with the knowledge of what they are financially due, allows healthcare facilities to bill correctly, and reduces claim denials or delays. Ensuring insurance coverage minimizes the cost of health services to patients.

Question: How does a patient intake process support effective care delivery?
Answer: During the process of patient intake, crucial info is collected about the patient, such as medical history, insurance details, and contact particulars. Such information enables healthcare providers to ease administrative processes, make informed decisions, and reduce errors in the care of patients.

Question: Why is Communication Relevant to Health?
Answer: Effective healthcare can only be achieved through communication. It facilitates the sharing of crucial information between healthcare practitioners, patients, and their families. Good communication helps in the correct diagnosis, safe treatment, and satisfied patients. With poor communication, there may be misunderstandings, which could result in medical errors.

Question: Why would they ever schedule follow-up appointments?
Answer: Follow-up visits are essential for continuous patient care and follow-up. It enables healthcare providers to monitor the effectiveness of a patient's treatment, adjust as necessary, and support continuity of care. This ensures better results on the part of the patient, subsequently contributing to good health.

Question: What is the meaning of scope of practice?
Answer: It states the boundaries of a healthcare professional's tasks and responsibilities that they legally and ethically can perform. It is profession-specific and dependent on state laws, professional regulations, and training frameworks.

Question: What does PHI include?
Answer: This can incorporate the address, name of the patient, medical record number (MRN), health problems diagnosed from NAAT tests, and previous management procedures, among other PHI components

Question: How does a Certified Medical Assistant contribute to a team-based healthcare approach?
Answer: A Certified Medical Assistant (CMA) would connect many dots in team-based healthcare. They work with nurses, doctors, and other health professionals for effective care of patients. CMAs do jobs like vitals and preparing patients for exams and procedures; this enables other team members to concentrate on their core undertakings.

Question: How does active listening contribute to patient communication?
Answer: Patient communication involves active listening. This involves entirely focusing on what a patient is saying, understanding, and responding. This helps generate trust, establish open communication, and make healthcare providers understand a patient's concerns, thus leading to enhanced care.

Question: What is the primary purpose of a patient's medical record?
Answer: The primary purpose of a patient's medical record is to keep the diagnosis, treatment, and healthcare interactions as required. This is a legal and accurate health record of a patient's condition, which helps in diagnosis, treatment planning, and continuity of care.

Question: What is the significance of patient advocacy to medical assisting?
Answer: Medical assistant has a duty in patient advocacy. They help pass the patient's concerns and preferences to the healthcare team. They promote because they are involved in lobbying, advocating, and from the public to ensure that their rights, needs, and informed decisions are made.

Question: How can cultural competence improve healthcare delivery?
Answer: Cultural competence refers to appreciating the cultural backgrounds, beliefs, and values of people as clients. It contributes to the efficacy of healthcare delivery by promoting effective communication, trust, and shared understanding among healthcare providers and patients with various cultural backgrounds. This leads to a narrowing of the health gap and enhances patient results.

Question: What does patient discharge involve?
Answer: Patient discharge refers to letting a patient leave a healthcare facility. This includes appropriate post-care instructions, prescriptions, and follow-up appointments to ensure the patient is well-prepared for home-based self-care. The patient's safety relies on good discharge planning.

Question: What are some standard safety precautions taken in a healthcare environment?
Answer: Some of the standard safety precautions while in a medical premise are hand hygiene and ensuring one is on the correct PPE, which will include appropriate masks and gloves. Being able to follow infection procedures should be observed, including proper disposal of health facilities waste, good sterility, and cleanliness observance, as well as observing how equipment is constantly being used with care.

Question: What does the term "patient-centered care" mean?
Answer: Patient-centered care is an approach that places the patient at the center of their healthcare. It involves tailoring care to patients' needs, preferences, and values. It emphasizes collaboration, communication, and shared decision-making between patients and healthcare providers.

Question: What is one of the primary responsibilities of a Certified Medical Assistant in managing prescriptions?
Answer: One of the critical responsibilities of a Certified Medical Assistant in prescription management is recording and passing accurate data to pharmacies. They may provide medicine, dosages, and instructions as directed by health providers to patients.

Question: How do communication adequacy and patient satisfaction relate?
Answer: Good communication is vital to patient satisfaction since it supports comprehension, confidence, and empathy. Patients with efficient communication feel listened to and provided with information and will be part of the decision-making regarding their care. This also leads to reduced miscommunication aimed at enhancing general patients' experiences.

Question: Literature and "Do Not Resuscitate" (DNR) order in healthcare.
Answer: Do Not Resuscitate order, a legal directive to healthcare givers not to apply cardiopulmonary resuscitation (CPR) on a patient who has suffered either cardiac arrest or respiratory arrest. That means it should respect a patient's living will.

Question: The principle of beneficence in medical ethics: what does it mean?
Answer: Corners of medical ethics, for example, include the principle of beneficence that stipulates the patient's best interests. It embodies care that meets the patient's health, risk elimination, and outcome optimization.

Question: What Makes the "Five Rights" of Medication Administration Vital in Healthcare?
Answer: Core to reducing medication errors within a healthcare facility, the "Five Rights" of medication administration (right patient, right drug, correct dose, correct route, and patient's rights to refuse treatment or medicine). These rights improve patient safety, minimize adverse events, and support proper medication administration.

Question: Explain Informed Consent in Medical Procedures.
Answer: Informed consent is when a patient chooses to undergo a medical procedure/ treatment with full knowledge. This involves providing the patient with information on a system, its risks and benefits, and alternatives and allowing autonomous decisions.

Question: How Does the HITECH Act and EHRs Fit?
Answer: The HITECH Act and EHRs: Stimulating the Adoption of Electronic Health Records and the Meaningful Use of Health Information Technology. It provides monetary incentives for the adoption of EHRs by medical practitioners whose main aim is to improve healthcare, efficiency in practice, and data storage.

Question: What is the Role of the Clinical Laboratory Improvement Amendments (CLIA) in healthcare, and how does it impact laboratory testing?
Answer: CLIA refers to a federal law that governs the laboratory testing process to guarantee its results' accuracy and reliability. This sets the standard for laboratories, proficiency testing, and certification requirements to ensure quality and safety in laboratory testing in healthcare.

Question: To what extent does the Health Insurance Portability and Accountability Act (HIPAA) address the privacy and security of patient health information?
Answer: The main reasons for its implementation are to protect patient's privacy and ensure the safety of health information. It establishes the benchmark for secure transmission and storage of Protected Health Information (PHI), regulates access to patient data, and compels occurrence reporting. HIPAA ensures the medical record and patient's confidentiality.

Question: Describe what medical malpractice is and how caregivers can reduce their liability risk.
Answer: Medical malpractice is simply the negligence or inappropriate exercise of power by a professional person about his employment. Simple measurements will enable health providers to keep low and manageable risks by accurately documenting care, obtaining informed consent, maintaining good professional standards, and having insurance for their profession.

Question: What is the impact of the National Practitioner Data Bank (NPDB) on healthcare providers, and what purpose does NPDB have in healthcare?
Answer: The NPDB maintains a database of information regarding the competence and conduct of healthcare professionals. It is a tool that hospitals and other healthcare institutions can use to determine the credentials of potential employees/providers. Its Role is to keep up the standards of HSMPs in healthcare professionals.

Question: What Does Stark Law Do With Compliance Programs in Tertiary Care Teaching Hospitals?
Answer: This Stark Law is intended to deter self-referral and financial relationships that may encourage overusing healthcare services. This law prohibits physicians from referring patients for only designated health services in entities they have a financial relationship with unless there is an exception.

Question: Discuss medical ethics committees in health care institutions and their Role in addressing ethical dilemmas.
Answer: It comprises healthcare professionals, administrators, and ethicists who address ethical issues, considering that all issues touching life are dealt with here. They guide, consult, and recommend appropriate courses of action in these instances, bearing ethical principles and legal considerations in mind.

Question: What is the Role of the Centers for Medicare & Medicaid Services (CMS) in the U.S. healthcare system?
Answer: CMS refers to the Centers for Medicare and Medicaid Services, the governing body for federal health-related initiatives. It sets the standards for health services and manages health data and payment systems to improve accessibility and quality of care.

Question: Describe the critical Roles of a Medical Office Administrator in a Health Practice.
Answer: A Medical Office Administrator supervises administrative activities in a medical office. This includes making appointments, handling bills, checking for insurance, and other administrative activities to make the front office run smoothly. They provide innumerable benefits to patient satisfaction and practice efficiency.

Question: Describe the Role of the Agency for Healthcare Research and Quality in improving patient safety and quality of care.
Answer: Agency for healthcare research and Quality, Evidence on the best practice proof in Health Care Safety. It enables healthcare providers to encourage best practices and assists in the minimization of medical errors and better patient outcomes.

Question: Demonstrate the Medical home model of healthcare for better patient care.
Answer: One model that focuses on coordinated and proper care is a Patient-centered Home Model. It helps provide care by coordinating care and enabling prevention and patient involvement, a single point of contact for healthcare.

Question: What is the Role of the FDA in Regulating Healthcare Products to Ensure They Are Safe?
Answer: The FDA (Food and Drug Administration) regulates the safety of food, drugs, medical devices, and other healthcare products in the United States. The FDA conducts pre-market evaluations, post-market surveillance, and enforcement of the law to ensure the public's safety towards products and drugs.

Question: How Is the Controlled Substances Act, and how are the Drugs Classified or Regulated?
Answer: The Controlled Substances Act of 1970 categorizes and regulates addictive drugs and substances. This defines substances into schedules based on their medical application and potential for abuse; it puts in place stringent controls over the manufacture, distribution, and prescription of such drugs.

Question: What are the ethical considerations surrounding end-of-life care and advanced directives?
Answer: Advanced Directives for End-of-Life Care incorporate ethically related concerns to end-of-life care, euthanasia, and provisions for respecting wishes. The health care providers may as well uphold these directives, including do-not-resuscitate (DNR) orders or living wills, ensuring that they also consider what is best for this patient.

Question: Explain the Role Of the Clinical Nurse Specialist (CNS) in the Healthcare Team and Contributions to the Quality of Patient Care.
Answer: The Clinical Nurse Specialist (CNS) is an advanced practice nurse specializing in a particular patient population or clinical area. For instance, specialist nurses are involved in patient care, act as clinicians in their area of specialization, and translate clinical know-how into education, evidence-based practice 'EBP,' research, and leadership, which yield better patient outcomes.

Question: Explain the Awareness, benefits, and challenges of telehealth depending upon delivery.
Answer: Telehealth is defined as the application of technology in providing healthcare services over a distance. Its effect affects healthcare delivery because it extends care, shortens travel distance, and provides convenience to the doorstep. The benefits involved better access, although technology limiting and privacy issues were challenging.

Question: How Does the Certified Professional Coder (CPC) Help Accurately Bill and code?
Answer: Codes for medical diagnoses and procedures relating to billing for payment are assigned by a Certified Professional Coder (CPC). They assist in facilitating accurate medical billing through proper coding, keeping up with all coding guidelines, and relaying relevant healthcare provider information to payers.

Question: What is patient engagement, and what are its clinical implications?
Answer: Patient engagement refers to patients' counseling themselves into health care and treatment decisions. Enhancing adherence to treatment plans, self-care, and health in general leads to better healthcare outcomes. They engage patients in health and healthcare, resulting in optimal health and reduced costs.

Question: How Do Healthcare Organizations Strive to Achieve Cultural Competence to Available Care for the Diverse Patient Populations?
Answer: Healthcare organizations attain cultural competency by providing training and education to their health professionals, having a diverse workforce, and offering care that meets the cultural, linguistic, and religious needs of patients from different populations. This enables equal treatment for all patients.

Question: What is the Role of the Medical Administrative Assistant in managing patient appointments, and how do they optimize the scheduling process?
Answer: A Medical Administrative Assistant coordinates patient appointments, designs the schedule to reduce wait times, and efficiently uses care providers' time. By managing the appointment process well, they aid in patient satisfaction and practice efficiency.

Question: What is the "Patient Bill of Rights" protecting patients in health care, and what would be its essential part?
Answer: The Patients' Bill of Rights contains the rights and responsibilities of the patient in care. This protects the patients by ensuring they are treated respectfully, obtaining informed consent, keeping their privacy, and participating in their care decisions. It enhances patient-centered care and the Autonomy of patients.

Question: How does the Health Resources and Services Administration (HRSA) address access to care for underserved populations?
Answer: HRSA is committed to improving access in underserved populations. This is achieved by providing funds to healthcare centers, increasing the health workforce, and combating healthcare disparities to guarantee that vulnerable and underserved communities' needs for quality care are met.

Question: How do healthcare organizations apply the principles of ethical decision-making when faced with such complex cases as resource alacrity in a critical situation?
Answer: In this regard, healthcare organizations sustain ethical decision-making guidelines and frameworks for the transparent distribution of resources, especially during crisis times. They consider things such as a patient's need for it and the benefits that a patient will potentially get from it based on medical criteria while observing ethical principles like justice, fairness, and transparency.

Question: What ethical concerns arise from organ transplantation, and how are donors and recipients chosen?
Answer: The ethical issues in organ transplantation include equitable distribution of organs, informed consent, and protection from abuse. The selection of donors and recipients is guided by medical criteria, compatibility, the urgency of organ need, and waiting list status, the primary role being to save lives while at the same time abiding by ethical considerations.

Question: How Does the Healthcare Effectiveness Data and Information Set (HEDIS) Support Provider-Oriented Quality Improvement?
Answer: HEDIS is a set of performance measures used for validating the quality and performance of patients. It is central to standardizing data collection and furnishing benchmarks for healthcare quality improvement.

Question: What is the Role of the Clinical Laboratory Scientist (CLS) in the diagnostic process, and how do they ensure the accuracy of test results?
Answer: CLS diagnoses several illnesses carried out on a sample collected from a patient. They pay great attention to sample handling, quality control measures, and instrument maintenance and adhere closely to strict testing protocols to ensure accurate test results.

Question: What are "patient rights" about ethically sound healthcare practices, and what are the fundamental patient rights?
Answer: The essence of patient rights in ethical healthcare practices is safeguarding patients' Autonomy, dignity, and safety. For instance, inherent in a patient's rights are informed consent, privacy & confidentiality, and participation.

Question: Clinical nurse leader role in healthcare and improving patient care outcomes.
Answer: Clinical Nurse Leader (CNL) is an APN role focused on clinical leadership. They enhance patient care by coordinating care, managing resources, promoting evidence-based practice, and facilitating communication within the healthcare team.

Question: What are the effects of the Affordable Care Act on access to and coverage of healthcare, and what are some main provisions?
Answer: In the U.S., ACS enhanced healthcare accessibility and coverage by enlarging insurance choices, giving lower prices to eligible people, and increasing Medicaid. A few critical ones include pre-existing conditions, essential health benefits, and the individual mandate for insurance.

Question: Define Patient-Centered Medical Homes in Health Care and Explain How They Enhance Adult Patient Care.
Answer: Patient-centered medical homes work as healthcare delivery models that deliver coordinated and comprehensive care from the doctor's end. They improve the quality of patient care via enhanced access to care, better coordination of care, more emphasis on preventive services, and engagement of patients in their health.

What is confidentiality in the context of medical law and ethics?

Confidentiality in healthcare refers to the obligation of medical professionals to keep a patient's medical information private unless the patient gives explicit consent for specific information to be share**D.** This includes information transmitted verbally, as well as information stored in medical records or other documents. Confidentiality is a fundamental ethical and legal standard to promote trust and honesty between patients and healthcare providers.

What does PHI stand for?

PHI stands for Protected Health Information. This term is primarily used in the context of health information privacy and security in the United States, where it refers to any information about health status, provision of healthcare, or payment for healthcare that can be linked to a specific individual. This is interpreted broadly and includes any part of a patient's medical record or payment history.

Which legislation aims to protect patient privacy and sets rules about who can access health records?

The Health Insurance Portability and Accountability Act (HIPAA) is a federal law in the United States that aims to protect patient privacy. HIPAA sets strict rules about who can access health records and under what circumstances, ensuring that individuals' medical information is kept confidential and secure. Violations of HIPAA can result in severe penalties, including fines and imprisonment.

What is the primary goal of OSHA?

The Occupational Safety and Health Administration (OSHA), a U.S. government agency, aims to ensure that workers have safe and healthful working conditions. OSHA sets and enforces standards for workplace safety and health. It also provides training, outreach, education, and assistance to employers and employees to help them understand and comply with these standards.

Define autonomy in the context of medical ethics.

In medical ethics, autonomy refers to the right of patients to make informed decisions about their healthcare. It means that medical professionals must respect patients' decisions about their treatment, even if the professional disagrees with the decision. Autonomy is a crucial principle in medical ethics, reflecting respect for individual self-determination and freedom of choice.

What is an EMR?

An EMR, or Electronic Medical Record, is a digital version of a patient's traditional paper medical chart. An EMR contains a patient's medical history, diagnoses, medications, treatment plans, immunization dates, allergies, radiology images, and laboratory and test results. It can be created, managed, and consulted by authorized clinicians and staff within one healthcare organization.

What is a crucial advantage of stream scheduling in a medical setting?

Stream or fixed appointment scheduling is where each patient is given a specific appointment time. One of its key advantages is that it can lead to a predictable and smooth flow of patients through the office, minimizing waiting times and allowing for individualized care. However, it requires precise time management and coordination to avoid delays and backlogs.

What is essential when managing a patient's appointment schedule?

An important consideration when managing a patient's appointment schedule is ensuring that the patient has clear and accurate information about necessary preparations. This could include instructions to fast or to take certain medications before the appointment. Proper scheduling also requires flexibility to accommodate emergencies, cancellations, and reschedules.

How often should hand hygiene be performed in a medical setting?

A: Hand hygiene is crucial to infection control in a medical setting and should be performed frequently. It should be carried out before and after every patient interaction, before and after wearing gloves, after touching any potentially contaminated surfaces or objects, and after personal activities such as using the restroom or eating. Proper hand hygiene helps prevent the spread of infection and protect healthcare workers and patients.

What does PPE stand for in a medical context?

In a medical context, PPE stands for Personal Protective Equipment. This is equipment that healthcare workers wear to minimize exposure to hazards that cause workplace injuries and illnesses. PPE may include gloves, medical masks, respirators, goggles, face shields, and gowns. PPE is a vital part of infection control in healthcare settings.

Why is patient consent meaningful before performing any medical procedure?

Patient consent is crucial as it respects the patient's autonomy, their right to make informed decisions about their healthcare. Before any medical procedure, the healthcare provider must explain the benefits, risks, and alternatives to the patient. This allows the patient to understand what they consent to and ensures that their rights are upheld.

How does medical coding contribute to healthcare?

Medical coding is essential in healthcare by converting patient health information into standardized billing, research, and health planning codes. These codes ensure uniformity and accuracy and aid in reimbursement from insurance companies. Additionally, they provide valuable data for tracking health trends and managing healthcare resources.

What is the role of a Certified Medical Assistant in patient education?

A Certified Medical Assistant plays a vital role in patient education, explaining medical procedures, providing instructions for medications and self-care post-procedure, and answering patients' questions. This education aids in patient compliance, improves health outcomes, and increases patient satisfaction by helping them make informed decisions about their healthcare.

What is the significance of maintaining accurate patient records?

Maintaining accurate patient records is critical for numerous reasons. It provides a detailed history of a patient's healthcare, which aids in medical decision-making and continuity of care. Accurate records are also necessary for legal protection, auditing, research, and reimbursement.

Why is it important to verify insurance coverage for patients?

Verifying insurance coverage is an essential administrative task in healthcare settings. It ensures that the services provided are covered under the patient's insurance policy, which prevents unexpected costs for the patient and guarantees that the healthcare provider will receive payment for their services. This process also helps identify any necessary pre-authorizations or referrals.

How does a patient intake process ensure efficient care delivery?

The patient intake process, which involves gathering comprehensive information about a patient, is essential for efficient care delivery. It ensures healthcare providers have accurate and current information about a patient's health status, medical history, allergies, and medications, facilitating appropriate and personalized treatment planning.

What role does communication play in healthcare settings?

Communication is vital in healthcare settings. It facilitates collaboration between healthcare providers, ensuring continuity and coordination of care. Effective communication with patients improves health outcomes, patient satisfaction, and adherence to treatment plans. It also plays a role in educating patients about their health and treatments and reducing healthcare delivery errors.

What is the purpose of scheduling follow-up appointments?

Scheduling follow-up appointments is crucial to monitor a patient's progress, evaluating the effectiveness of treatments, make necessary adjustments to the care plan, and provide ongoing education and support. They also ensure that any complications or adverse reactions are promptly identified and addressed. These appointments contribute to continuity of care and help improve health outcomes.

What does the term "scope of practice" mean?

The term "scope of practice" refers to the activities a healthcare provider can perform based on their professional license, skills, and training. It outlines the procedures, actions, and processes the provider is competent and legally permitted to perform. Adhering to one's scope of practice ensures patient safety and quality of care.

What does PHI include?

PHI, or Protected Health Information, includes any health-related information that can be linked to an individual. This may encompass medical history, lab test results, diagnoses, treatment information, and billing information. PHI also includes demographic information like names, addresses, dates of birth, Social Security numbers, and other personal identifiers that could be used to identify the individual.

How does a Certified Medical Assistant contribute to a team-based healthcare approach?

Certified Medical Assistants contribute significantly to a team-based healthcare approach by serving as a bridge between doctors, nurses, and patients. They perform clinical and administrative tasks, ensuring smooth workflow in healthcare settings. Their roles can range from scheduling appointments to taking vital signs, all of which support patient care and the healthcare team's goals.

What is the role of active listening in patient communication?
Active listening in patient communication is vital to understanding a patient's needs, concerns, and experiences. It involves fully concentrating, understanding, responding, and remembering what is said. This engagement level helps build trust and rapport, encourages patients to share vital health information, and ensures that healthcare providers can make well-informed decisions about a patient's care.

What is the primary function of a patient's medical record?
The primary function of a patient's medical record is to document the care and services provided to a patient chronologically. This includes diagnosis, treatment plans, progress notes, medications, laboratory results, and other relevant health information. Medical records serve as a communication tool between healthcare providers, ensuring continuity of care and aiding in clinical decision-making.

What role does patient advocacy play in a medical assistant's duties?
Patient advocacy is crucial to a medical assistant's duties. Advocacy can include educating patients about their rights, helping them navigate the healthcare system, or acting as an intermediary between patients and other healthcare providers. By advocating for patients, medical assistants help ensure patients receive appropriate care, respect, and understanding.

How can cultural competence improve healthcare delivery?
Cultural competence, the ability to understand and respect cultural differences and to respond appropriately to different cultural contexts, can significantly improve healthcare delivery. It can help to eliminate health disparities, improve communication, increase patient engagement, and ultimately enhance health outcomes. Understanding a patient's cultural context can lead to more personalized, effective care.

What does patient discharge involve?
Patient discharge involves a comprehensive planning and communication process to transition a patient from one level of care to another, often from a hospital to home. This includes a clear outline of the patient's current health status, a detailed plan for further consideration, medication instructions, scheduling follow-up appointments, and providing necessary education or resources to the patient or caregiver.

What are some standard safety procedures in a medical setting?
Common safety procedures in a medical setting include maintaining clean and sterile environments, proper hand hygiene, correct use and disposal of sharps, and regular equipment maintenance. Ensuring personal protective equipment (PPE) is worn when needed and adhering to safety protocols for storing and administering medications are also crucial for maintaining safety.

What does the term "patient-centered care" mean?
Patient-centered care refers to healthcare that is respectful of and responsive to individual patient preferences, needs, and values. The patient's values guide all clinical decisions, ensuring that the patient remains central to the care process. This approach has improved patient satisfaction, health outcomes, and healthcare delivery efficiency.

What is one of the primary responsibilities of a Certified Medical Assistant in managing prescriptions?
One of the primary responsibilities of a Certified Medical Assistant in managing prescriptions is to facilitate clear communication between the doctor, patient, and pharmacy. This could involve preparing medicines for the doctor's signature, instructing patients on how and when to take their medication, and liaising with pharmacies to ensure that prescriptions are filled correctly.

How can adequate communication impact patient satisfaction?
Effective communication has a profound impact on patient satisfaction. Patients who feel heard, understood, and valued are more likely to be satisfied with their care. Effective communication can also lead to better health outcomes, as patients who understand their diagnosis and treatment plan are more likely to adhere to medical advice and engage in their healthcare.

CONCLUSION

As we draw the curtain on this comprehensive guide to the Certified Medical Assistant (CMA) certification, you have been equipped with an in-depth understanding of what it takes to be a top-notch CMA. The journey through the terrain of medical assistance is nuanced and multi-faceted, requiring an optimal blend of knowledge, dexterity, and professionalism. We hope this guide has not only offered ability but also stirred in you the passion needed to excel in this field.

Our exploration of the medical landscape, from clinical workflow to pharmacology, safety, infection control, medical laws, and ethics, has unveiled the diverse and complex responsibilities that await you as a CMA. It's an incredible journey where each day offers an opportunity to make a significant difference in the lives of patients and their families.

The healthcare field is an ever-evolving ecosystem requiring a constant hunger for learning. This book has shed light on the primary roles and responsibilities you'll take on as a CMA and the critical soft skills necessary for success, like communication and empathy. Remember, while your technical skills will get you in the door, these soft skills will keep you in the room.

Our coverage of regulatory guidelines and legal and ethical considerations is a compass in navigating the often complex healthcare legal environment. These guidelines are not just laws or recommendations; they are the standards that uphold the integrity of the healthcare profession.

To help solidify your understanding and evaluate your readiness for the CMA examination, we've included a series of practice tests, from clinical procedures to billing and coding. These questions, while challenging, offer a glimpse into the breadth and depth of the CMA exam and are meant to give you confidence as you embark on your certification journey.

Finally, we discussed the importance of health information management and appointment scheduling. In the modern healthcare system, the effective management of health information is not just a necessity; it is a lifeline that ensures the seamless operation of healthcare institutions.

This book represents the culmination of your journey toward becoming a Certified Medical Assistant, but in many ways, it's just the beginning. As you venture into the field, remember that every patient interaction, every lab result, and every appointment scheduled contributes to your growth as a healthcare professional and enriches the lives of those you serve.

As you close this book, open your mind to the infinite possibilities. We hope this guide is an indispensable tool for preparing for the CMA exam and a valuable resource throughout your healthcare career. Becoming a CMA is more than just a title; it is a commitment to service, excellence, and lifelong learning.

Welcome to the exciting, rewarding world of medical assistance! Here's to a future where every patient you encounter benefits from the skills, knowledge, and passion you bring to this noble profession.

SPECIAL EXTRA CONTENT

Congratulations on Completing This Educational Journey!

Dear esteemed reader, If these final words are resonating with you, it signifies that you have successfully navigated through a path of personal and professional development, and we are privileged to have been part of your journey towards knowledge.

Your Insights Are Invaluable!

Your experiences, reflections, and feedback on the material you've just completed are crucial to us. We earnestly encourage you to share your thoughts about our book on Amazon. Whether a particular section struck a chord with you or the overall journey through the pages has broadened your understanding, your perspective is immensely important. By sharing your experiences, you help guide other learners and provide us, the authors, with the inspiration needed to refine our work and continue delivering impactful content.

Uncover Special EXTRA CONTENT Reserved Just for You!

In appreciation of your commitment, we've prepared exclusive additional content specifically for our readers. Here's what awaits you:

- **MP3 audio files** for you to listen to whenever and wherever you want!
- An eBook titled "**Medical Terminology for Health Careers.**"
- **NOW +600 flashcards <u>with pictures</u>** featuring "**Medical Terms**" for quick recall and enhanced comprehension. **Note. FLASHCARDS ARE READY TO USE FOR FREE** online or offline! You can track your progress and conveniently and interactively memorize the most important terms and concepts! Download to your device: ***Anki APP or Anki Droid***, or enter the web page and register free of charge. Then import the files we have given you as a gift and use the flashcards whenever and wherever you want to study and track your progress.
- Digital version of this book
- **20** In-depth **Case Studies** offering real-world insights into patient safety, ethics, pain management, clinical communication, and care in varied settings.

Straightforward Resources for Ongoing Enrichment

Below, you will find a distinctive QR CODE leading directly to your bonus content, ready for immediate download and exploration. There's no need for email subscriptions or personal detail disclosures; this is our direct gift to you, supporting your continued educational journey seamlessly.

Should you encounter any issues or have any questions regarding the downloadable material, please feel free to reach out to us at **booklovers.1001@gmail.com**

Sending warm regards and best wishes for your future endeavors.
With heartfelt thanks!

We look forward to your feedback!
Thank you!

Made in the USA
Las Vegas, NV
31 May 2024